General Astrophysics

with Elements of Geophysics

General Astrophysics

with Elements of Geophysics

Jerzy S. Stodółkiewicz

Polish Academy of Sciences

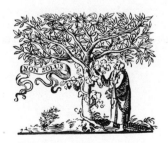

American Elsevier Publishing Company, Inc.

New York　　　　　London　　　　　Amsterdam

ORIGINALLY PUBLISHED AS
Astrofizyka ogólna
z elementami geofizyki

Translated by Eugene Lepa

AMERICAN ELSEVIER PUBLISHING COMPANY, INC.
52 Vanderbilt Avenue, New York, N.Y. 10017

ELSEVIER PUBLISHING COMPANY
335 Jan Van Galenstraat, P.O. Box 211
Amsterdam, The Netherlands

International Standard Book Number 0-444-40872-X

Library of Congress Card Number 76-148458

Printed in Poland (DRP)

Contents

Preface

This book is intended as a text for a one-semester course in general astrophysics and the elements of geophysics, with 45 hours of lectures. Such a concise approach to astronomy makes it incumbent upon the lecturer and textbook author to give compact treatment to the basic observational methods and the results they yield, while briefly presenting the principal theoretical conclusions arrived at in investigations of various types of astronomical objects. While taking conciseness of presentation as a starting point, I have nevertheless tried to give a reasonably profound explanation of the causes, relations, and effects of physical phenomena occurring on astronomical objects. Consequently, careful selection of the material presented has been necessary and (to avoid repetition) more detailed discussion has been limited to typical representatives of the particular classes of celestial bodies.

The entire text has been divided into seven chapters. The first is a survey of fundamental observational methods and instruments. Chapter II is devoted to a discussion of those classical problems of the kinetics of the Earth which must be mastered for an understanding of the rest of the book. Subsequent chapters go into particular types of astronomical objects—the solar system, stars, galaxies, ending with cosmologies that treat the Universe as a whole. The properties of these objects are presented by referring to the best observed representatives of a given type as examples. The book therefore gives extensive treatment to the Earth, the Sun, and the Milky Way as examples of planets, stars and galaxies, respectively.

Although the textbook is addressed in principle to physics students, it may serve as supplementary reading for first-year astronomy courses and may also prove useful to amateur astronomers with an appropriate mathematical background.

The author wishes to take this opportunity to thank Professors Stefan Piotrowski and Włodzimierz Zonn for the suggestions and encouragement they provided during the writing of this book. Thanks are also due Dr. Krzysztof Serkowski for his critical appraisal of the entire manuscript and for a number of important suggestions, particularly in regard to Chapter I.

J.S.S.

Warsaw, August 1966

Preface to English Edition

This edition contains a number of additions and modifications introduced in order to take account of results obtained in this area of astronomy since publication of the Polish edition.

J.S.S.

Warsaw, December 1969

Introduction

The object of astronomy, as of physics, is to study the forms in which matter occurs, to investigate processes which take place in matter, and to discover the general laws governing those processes. There is a basic difference, however, between the methods of investigation used in physics and astronomy. The physicist can artifically reproduce in the laboratory most of the processes under study. While performing an experiment, one can (to a great extent) avoid side effects and control the conditions of the matter under study so that they facilitate learning about the phenomenon of interest. The astronomer has no such possibility. The first experimental work in astronomy began only recently with the utilization of space vehicles to take instruments into the proximity of near astronomical objects or with the transmission of radio signals emitted from the Earth and bounced off the surface of nearby objects. But despite the rapid advances made, these methods of investigation can be used only for the closest objects in the solar planetary system. In the overwhelming majority of cases the astronomer must still confine himself to observations, utilizing information contained in electromagnetic radiation, corpuscular cosmic radiation, or meteorites which reach the Earth. Thus, observation continues to be the fundamental method of astronomical research.

The differences between astronomy and physics, however, do not lie solely in methods of research. Differences also exist in the very essence of the object under study. Matter studied by the astronomer is under natural conditions, not under conditions produced in the laboratory. The phenomena which occur are observed without interference in their course. Many processes extant in nature cannot be reproduced in the laboratory because of the exceptional conditions required, such as extreme temperatures or densities of matter, large masses or enormous energies which are indispensable if these processes are to occur.

Precisely because of these differences, astronomy and physics are sciences which complement each other. Each provides problems which can be solved only with the active participation of the other. Collaboration between astronomers and physicists provides an opportunity for checking the applicability of the laws governing matter over the full range of conditions to be found in nature.

Chapter 1 Astronomical Observations

THE FUNDAMENTALS OF VISIBLE RADIATION

The richest source of information about astronomical objects is their electromagnetic radiation which reaches the Earth. For centuries only part of that radiation—radiation which produces visual sensations in man—was utilized in astronomical investigations. Only when radio engineering developed did it become possible to measure radio-frequency radiation, while rocket-borne instruments enabled studies to be made on wavelengths which are absorbed by the Earth's atmosphere.

Section 1 Light as Waves

Wave theory must be used to describe many properties of light (this will be the name employed here for the whole spectrum of electromagnetic radiation, not only the visible portion). According to this theory, light is a disturbance of electromagnetic field propagated in all directions from a point source. This disturbance is propagated as a wave causing the local electric and magnetic field to oscillate perpendicularly to each other and to the direction of propagation.

Variations in the electric field intensity can be described by the equation:

$$\mathbf{E} = \mathbf{E}_0 \cos\left[\frac{2\pi}{T}\left(t - \frac{x}{c}\right) + \delta\right], \qquad (1\text{-}1)$$

where $\mathbf{E}_0$, T, c, are constants, t denotes time, and x is the spatial coordinate measured in the direction of light propagation. The corresponding equation for the magnetic vector is of the form

$$\mathbf{H} = \mathbf{H}_0 \cos\left[\frac{2\pi}{T}\left(t - \frac{x}{c}\right) + \delta\right], \qquad (1\text{-}2)$$

where $\mathbf{H}_0 \perp \mathbf{E}_0$ and $\mathbf{E}_0 \perp \mathbf{i}_x$, $\mathbf{H}_0 \perp \mathbf{i}_x$, while $\mathbf{i}_x$ is the versor or unit vector along the x-axis.

Equations (1-1) and (1-2) describe the electric and magnetic vector vibrations propagated as plane waves of amplitudes $|\mathbf{E}_0|$ and $|\mathbf{H}_0|$, respectively. The argument of the cosine function in these equations,

$$\frac{2\pi}{T}\left(t - \frac{x}{c}\right) + \delta, \qquad (1\text{-}3)$$

is called the phase of the wave. Expression (1-3) remains constant when

$$x = ct \qquad (1\text{-}4)$$

which means that the phases of waves described by Eqs. (1-1) and (1-2) travel with a speed of c. This speed is 2.997925×10^{10} cm $\cdot$ sec^{-1} ($\approx 3 \times \times 10^{10}$ cm $\cdot$ sec^{-1}) *in vacuo* and is known as the speed of light. The constant δ specifies the initial phase (this is the phase at point $x = 0$ at the instant $t = 0$). The time T taken by electric (magnetic) vector vibrations to re-appear at the same point in space in the same phase—termed the period of the wave—is the last constant in Eqs. (1-1) and (1-2). Instead of the period, we shall use the frequency ν (number of oscillations per second):

$$\nu = T^{-1}, \qquad (1\text{-}5)$$

or the wavelength λ. The wavelength is the distance between two consecutive points on the x-axis, in the same phase. Since, by this definition, it is the path travelled by light in one period, the wavelength is uniquely related to the period and frequency by the formulae

$$\lambda = cT \qquad (1\text{-}6)$$

and

$$\lambda\nu = c. \qquad (1\text{-}7)$$

The propagation of a wave described by Eq. (1-1) is shown in Fig. 1-1.

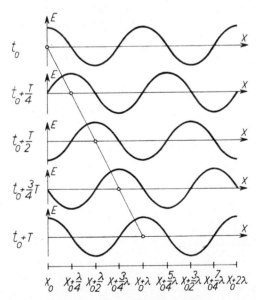

Figure 1-1. Propagation of a light wave. The magnitude of the electric vector is plotted against the distance x from the source of light, at intervals of a quarter-period. The inclined line connects points with the same phase.

· The electric vector could also vibrate in a fixed plane (vector **E** does not change direction) or the vibration plane may change. In the first case we speak of linearly polarized radiation. It is this case which is described by Eq. (1-1). The plane in which the electric vector vibrates is called the plane of polarization.

Section 2   Interference of Light Waves

Now let us consider the effects caused by the superposition—interference—of two electromagnetic waves of the same wavelength λ. First we shall examine the case when the electric vectors in both waves vibrate in the same direction. The resultant vibrations of the electric vector are described by the equation

$$E = E_{01} \cos\left[\frac{2\pi}{T}\left(t - \frac{x}{c}\right) + \delta_1\right] + E_{02} \cos\left[\frac{2\pi}{T}\left(t - \frac{x}{c}\right) + \delta_2\right], \quad (1\text{-}8)$$

where E_{01}, E_{02}, and δ_1, δ_2 are, respectively, the amplitudes and phases of both component waves.

Simple manipulation brings Eq. (1-8) to the form

$$E = E_0 \cos\left[\frac{2\pi}{T}\left(t - \frac{x}{c}\right) + \gamma\right], \quad (1\text{-}9)$$

where

$$E_0 \cos\gamma = E_{01} \cos\delta_1 + E_{02} \cos\delta_2, \quad (1\text{-}10)$$

$$E_0 \sin\gamma = E_{01} \sin\delta_1 + E_{02} \sin\delta_2. \quad (1\text{-}11)$$

If the component waves are in the same phase, i.e.

$$\delta_1 = \delta_2 = \delta \quad (1\text{-}12)$$

then, as implied by Eqs. (1-10) and (1-11),

$$\gamma = \delta, \quad (1\text{-}13)$$

$$E_0 = E_{01} + E_{02} \quad (1\text{-}14)$$

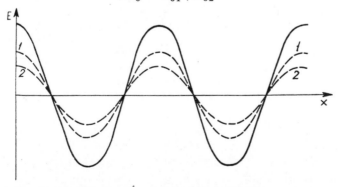

Figure 1-2. Interference of two waves of equal period and phase. - - component waves, — resultant wave.

which means that the resultant wave is in the same phase as the component waves, and its amplitude is equal to the sum of the amplitudes of the component waves. Superposition of the two waves has resulted in reinforcement of the radiation. This situation is illustrated in Fig. 1-2.

When the component waves differ in phase by 180°,

$$\delta_1 = \delta_2 + 180° = \delta \tag{1-15}$$

we have

$$\gamma = \delta, \tag{1-16}$$

$$E_0 = E_{01} - E_{02}. \tag{1-17}$$

Here we have wave attenuation (Cf. Fig. 1-3) or even complete destructive interference when $E_{01} = E_{02}$. In the latter case, light is not propagated in the medium (Fig. 1-4). In other cases we have various degrees of reinforcement or attenuation of waves.

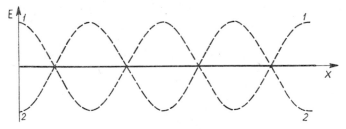

Figure 1-3. Interference of two waves of equal period, but with a phase difference of 180° between them. - - component waves, — resultant wave.

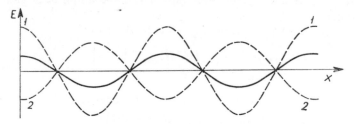

Figure 1-4. Destructive interference of two waves of equal period and amplitude, but with a phase difference of 180° between them.

Section 3 Polarization of Light

Different effects are produced, however, when the electric vectors of the waves superimposed do not vibrate in the same direction.

Without restricting the generality of the considerations, we may assume that the directions of the electric vector vibration in the two waves are perpendicular to each other. Indeed, if this were not so we could resolve each of the waves into two Y and Z components in which vibrations occur along two axes, Y and Z, at right angles to each other. Interference of the Y components of the two waves results in a wave in which the vibrations occur along the Y axis. A similar situation occurs for the Z components. Thus, a pair of linearly polarized waves, whose polarization planes are at a nonzero angle to each other, can be replaced by a pair of waves polarized in mutually perpendicular planes.

Let the component waves be of the form

$$\mathbf{E}_i = \mathbf{E}_{0i}\cos\left[\frac{2\pi}{T}\left(t - \frac{x}{c}\right) + \delta_i\right] \quad \text{for} \quad i = 1, 2, \quad (1\text{-}18)$$

where the vectors are

$$\mathbf{E}_{01} = [0, E_{01}, 0], \quad (1\text{-}19)$$

$$\mathbf{E}_{02} = [0, 0, E_{02}]. \quad (1\text{-}20)$$

These two waves are superimposed and, consequently, the electric vector vibrations will be represented by the equation

$$\mathbf{E} = \mathbf{E}_1 + \mathbf{E}_2$$

$$= \left[0, E_{01}\cos\left\{\frac{2\pi}{T}\left(t - \frac{x}{c}\right) + \delta_1\right\}, E_{02}\cos\left\{\frac{2\pi}{T}\left(t - \frac{x}{c}\right) + \delta_2\right\}\right]. \quad (1\text{-}21)$$

In cases when $\delta_1 = \delta_2 = \delta$ or $\delta_1 = \delta_2 + 180° = \delta$, Eq. (1-21) can be rewritten more simply as

$$\mathbf{E} = [0, E_{01}, \pm E_{02}]\cos\left[\frac{2\pi}{T}\left(t - \frac{x}{c}\right) + \delta\right]. \quad (1\text{-}22)$$

The direction of the electric vector vibrations $[0, E_{01}, \pm E_{02}]$ is fixed in both cases, which means that the light remains linearly polarized.

In all other cases the end of the electric vector describes an ellipse in the YZ plane. Light is then said to be elliptically polarized (Fig. 1-5).

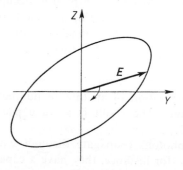

Figure 1-5. Electric vector vibrations of elliptically polarized light.

Circular polarization is a special case of elliptical polarization. This is produced by superposition of two waves (linearly polarized in two perpendicular planes) with the same amplitudes $E_{01} = E_{02} = E_0$ and phases differing by 90° ($\delta_1 = \delta_2 + 90° = \delta$ or $\delta_1 = \delta_2 - 90° = \delta$). For circularly polarized radiation (Fig. 1-6)

$$\mathbf{E} = \mathbf{E}_0 \left[0, \cos\left\{\frac{2\pi}{T}\left(t - \frac{x}{c}\right) + \delta\right\}, \ \mp\sin\left\{\frac{2\pi}{T}\left(t - \frac{x}{c}\right) + \delta\right\} \right]. \quad (1\text{-}23)$$

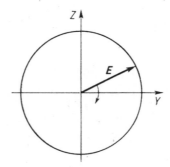

Figure 1-6. Electric vector vibrations of circularly polarized light.

Our discussion to this point has been based on acceptance of the wave theory of light. However, not all properties of light can be accounted for by this theory. We have seen, for instance, that the superposition of two (or more) linearly polarized waves yields waves which are also polarized (linearly or elliptically); we cannot in this way explain how unpolarized light comes into being. Nor is the photoelectric effect explicable in terms of wave theory. To elucidate these effects we resort to the corpuscular theory of light which treats light as an assemblage of particles—photons—moving through space at a velocity c. Each photon is indivisible, i.e. it must be either completely absorbed or completely transmitted by a medium. Moreover, a photon occupies a particular location in space whereas a wave, constituting an exactly periodic phenomenon, is infinitely extended. Indeed, light "signals" emitted by a source of light are bounded in space and time and, hence, are not an exactly periodic phenomenon.

This kind of wave motion occurring in only part of space, can be obtained by assuming the superposition of an infinite number of waves with only slightly differing periods. The result is a wave packet, which is shown graphically in Fig. 1-7.

Wave packets or photons propagate through space like particles, but retain wave properties (for instance, they have a capacity for interference). Natural (unpolarized) light consists of many packets of linearly or elliptically polarized waves with random directions of polarization. The phenomenon of polarization consists in a given flux containing only photons with one particular plane of polarization.

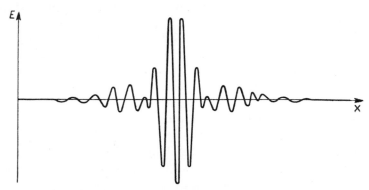

Figure 1-7. A wave packet.

Depending on the type of phenomenon discussed, we shall employ either the wave or the corpuscular theory of light. This also applies to the terminology: for instance, we shall speak of a light wave of frequency ν, or of a photon possessing energy E when referring to one and the same light radiation for which

$$E = h\nu, \qquad (1\text{-}24)$$

where $h = 6.62 \times 10^{-27}$ erg · sec is Planck's constant.

Section 4   Spectral Distribution

Radiation which lends itself to description as a set of waves having one particular frequency ν, or else as a beam of photons with the same energy E, is said to be monochromatic. In reality, all astronomical objects emit radiation of various frequencies. Part of this radiation, characterized by wavelengths between 4000 Å and 7500 Å (1 Å $= 10^{-8}$ cm), causes visual sensations in man. Radiation with wavelengths in this range is called visible radiation. All other radiation can be recorded only by means

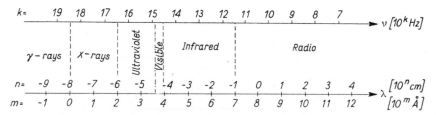

Figure 1-8. The electromagnetic spectrum.

of special apparatus suited to the purpose. Extending into the region of wavelengths shorter than visible radiation is ultraviolet radiation (4000 Å–100 Å), followed by X-rays, and gamma rays. Wavelengths longer than those of visible radiation are infrared (7500 Å–1 mm) and radio radiation. A schematic division of the electromagnetic spectrum is given in Fig. 1-8.

Section 5   Observed Features of Visible Radiation

The brief description of the properties of electromagnetic radiation in the preceding sections provides a basis for a survey of those properties of radiation which can be observed directly with astronomical instruments. All information about astronomical objects contained in the light radiation emitted by these objects must be obtained from the electromagnetic oscillations composing that radiation. This is why astronomical observations consist in measuring those properties of electromagnetic field oscillations which can be recorded by means of available apparatus.

The first such property, the one observed earliest, is the direction from which the radiation arrives. This is the name we shall give the direction of the unit vector

$$\mathbf{i} = \frac{\mathbf{E} \times \mathbf{H}}{|\mathbf{E} \times \mathbf{H}|}. \tag{1-25}$$

The direction of the unit vector **i** can be specified by a pair of numbers in some arbitrary coordinate system. The spherical coordinate system is the one used most frequently in astronomy. In this system each direction **i** is determined by two angles U and V. U is the angle between the perpendicular projection of the unit vector **i** onto a plane P (known as the principal or reference plane of the system) and a direction **k** (the reference direction of the system) which lies on plane P; while V is the angle between the unit vector **i** and the plane P (Cf. Fig. 1-9).

The measurement of the direction of radiation received provides us with partial information about the position of the luminous object. In-

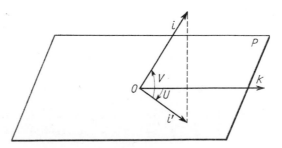

Figure 1-9. The spherical coordinate system.

formation sufficient to specify positions of celestial objects includes distance determinations in addition to angle. (See, for example, the discussion of trigonometrical parallax as a method of distance determination in Sec. 15). Several measurements performed at some specified interval of time enable us to draw conclusions about the motion of the source of light relative to the observer.

Another characteristic of radiation which reaches us is the illumination $\mathscr{E}$. This is the amount of energy per unit time incident on a unit area of surface perpendicular to the direction of the radiation. The illumination is determined by the amplitudes of the oscillations performed by the electric and magnetic vectors since they are the vectors which determine the energy of wave motion. By the definition above the unit of illumination is erg $\cdot$ cm$^{-2} \cdot$ sec^{-1}. Later we shall also use the concept of luminous flux which is defined as the amount of luminous energy per unit time incident on a surface (the unit of flux is erg $\cdot$ sec^{-1}) and the luminous intensity I, defined as the amount of energy emitted into a unit solid angle by a source per unit time (the unit of luminous intensity is erg $\cdot$ sec$^{-1} \cdot$ $\cdot$ steradian^{-1}). The illumination from radiation reaching the observer depends on the amount of energy (per unit time) emitted by the source of light, on the distance of the source from the observer, and on the optical properties (scattering, absorption) of the medium through which the light must travel. For this reason illumination measurements provide us with information about the distance of astronomical objects, the energy conditions on these objects, and the matter present in the space which the light ray has traversed.

No one astronomical instrument enables us to measure illumination at all wavelengths. Each astronomical instrument is designed for radiation from a particular spectral range. For this reason, the value of illumination obtained by a single measurement determines only the energy of radiation received in a particular range of the spectrum. This situation, however, is not disadvantageous since several measurements by a suitably chosen set of instruments informs us about the distribution of radiation in various parts of the spectrum. We then speak of illumination in particular colours.

The next question is: what is the distribution of the incident radiation as a function of the wavelength? To find the answer to this question, the beam of incident light must be directed at an optical system with different properties for each wavelength. Upon passing through such a system, radiation of various wavelengths can be recorded independently. In this case we speak of the spectral distribution of the radiation under study. It is evident from the above that the spectral distribution is specified if for a given radiation we give a function

$$\mathscr{E}(\lambda) \tag{1-26}$$

defined as the limit, as $\Delta\lambda$ tends to zero, of the ratio of the illumination of the radiation with wavelengths in the interval $[\lambda, \lambda+\Delta\lambda]$ to the width of that interval, $\Delta\lambda$. The unit used here is $\mathrm{erg\cdot cm^{-2}\cdot sec^{-1}\cdot \mathring{A}^{-1}}$. Of course

$$\int_0^\infty \mathscr{E}(\lambda)d\lambda = \mathscr{E}, \qquad (1\text{-}27)$$

where $\mathscr{E}$ is the total illumination.

In addition to gradual changes of illumination with wavelength (continuous spectrum), lines and bands (band spectrum) occur in the radiation spectrum of astronomical objects (Cf. Plate 1)*.

The energy distribution in a continuous spectrum depends on the temperature of the radiating body (in general, hotter bodies emit radiation which has its maximum in a range of shorter wavelength region than the maximum of radiation from cooler bodies). Light in various parts of the spectrum is attenuated in varying degree as it travels through a scattering medium (in general, more strongly for shorter waves). The result is that objects observed through a layer of interstellar matter appear redder than they are in actual fact. This is why observations of the continuous spectrum provide us with information about the temperature of the radiating body, as well as about the thickness and optical properties of the scattering medium interposed between the object and the observer. Every gas radiates and absorbs a set of spectral lines specific to it. Comparison of the observed spectrum with the arrays of spectral lines obtained in the laboratory for various gases enables us to determine the chemical composition of the radiating object. The shape of the spectral lines (Fig. 1-10)

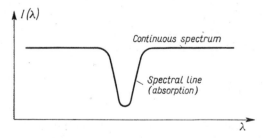

Figure 1-10. Shape of a spectral line. Distribution of illumination as a function of wavelength.

and the ratios of their intensities are functions of the pressure and temperature of the given object. When radiation passes through a medium which is not altogether transparent, absorption lines characteristic of that

---

* All the plates are at the end of the book.

medium appear in the spectrum. This yields further information about the matter interposed between the radiation-emitting astronomical object and the observer.

The positions of lines in the observed spectrum also depend on the motion of the observer and light source relative to each other. If the observer and light source move with respect to each other at a speed such that the radial component is v_r, the observed frequency will be changed by Δv with respect to the emitted frequency v, in keeping with the Doppler effect formula

$$\frac{\Delta v}{v} = -\frac{v_r}{c}. \tag{1-28}$$

The Doppler effect provides the main source of information about the radial velocities of astronomical objects.

Finally, the last observed feature of radiation is its polarization. In order to detect polarization, the incident radiation is directed into a polarizer. This is an instrument capable of loss-free (theoretically) transmission of radiation which is linearly polarized in some plane and complete absorption of radiation which is polarized perpendicular to that plane. If unpolarized radiation arrives from the object under study, the intensity of the light ray leaving the polarizer does not depend on the orientation of the polarizer (Fig. 1-11). On the other hand, if the incident light is

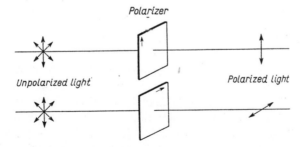

Figure 1-11. Passage of unpolarized light through a polarizer.

linearly polarized, the intensity of the radiation leaving the polarizer will be a function of the polarizer orientation and will change from I to 0 (Fig. 1-12) as the polarizer is turned. In practice, the radiation from astronomical objects is partially polarized, which means that as the polarizer is turned, the intensity varies from a maximum value $I_{\max}$ to a minimum value $I_{\min} > 0$. The ratio

$$p = \frac{I_{\max} - I_{\min}}{I_{\max} + I_{\min}} \tag{1-29}$$

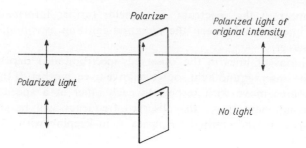

Figure 1-12. Passage of polarized light through a polarizer.

is called the degree of polarization and is usually expressed in per cent. The direction of polarization can be determined from the orientation of the polarizer in a position such that the intensity of the radiation transmitted is a maximum I_{max}.

Light is polarized as a result of optical anisotropy in the radiating medium, or in the medium between the light source and the observer. Consequently, polarization measurements are a source of information about the factors which cause this anisotropy.

All of the aforementioned features of radiation from astronomical objects may be stable or may be subject to variations with time which are indicative of changes occurring on luminous objects and possibly in the medium between the light source and the observer.

Section 6   The Influence of the Earth's Atmosphere on Astronomical Observation

The presence of the atmosphere distorts the results of astronomical observations made from the Earth's surface. Owing to refraction of light in the atmosphere, the direction from which the radiation arrives does not in general coincide with the actual direction of the source of light. Scattering and absorption of radiation in the atmosphere reduce the observed brightness of astronomical objects. Finally, air movement and turbulence distort the images obtained. The terrestrial atmosphere is completely opaque in some regions of the electromagnetic spectrum. Observations in these spectral regions cannot be made from the Earth's surface. Hence, the introduction of instruments into rockets and space vehicles travelling beyond the Earth's atmosphere has been extremely important for the development of astronomical research.

Electromagnetic radiation is subject to absorption, scattering, and reflection as it traverses the atmosphere. This phenomenon is known as atmospheric extinction. The transparency of the atmosphere as well as the magnitude of extinction depends on the wavelength of the incident radiation. In the visible region, for instance, the transparency of the atmosphere is about 80% (i.e. the ratio of intensity of the transmitted radiation to that of the radiation incident perpendicular to the atmosphere is about 0.8), but decreases for shorter wavelengths and in the infrared. The atmosphere is completely opaque in some regions of the spectrum. Radiation of wavelengths shorter than 3000 Å is completely absorbed by ozone (Cf. Sec. 24) and by the ionosphere (Cf. Sec. 26). The infrared—radiation of wavelengths from about 20,000 Å to about 1 mm—is absorbed by water vapour (Cf. Sec. 24). And, finally, radio waves longer than about 20 m are reflected off the upper layers of the ionosphere (Cf. Sec. 26). The Earth's atmosphere transmits (Cf. Fig. 1-13) only radiation whose

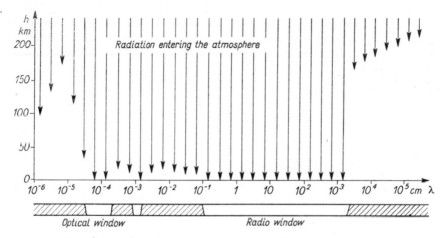

Figure 1-13. Transmission of radiation through the atmosphere; atmospheric windows.

wavelengths lie in the interval 3000 Å $< \lambda <$ 20,000 Å (the so-called atmospheric window—visible radiation comes within this interval), some infrared radiation (8×10^{-4} cm $< \lambda < 1.3 \times 10^{-3}$ cm), and radio waves with wavelengths ranging from about 1 mm to about 20 mm (radio window).

ASTRONOMICAL INSTRUMENTS

The object of astronomical observations is to record or measure, as accurately as possible, the actual values of parameters which characterize one or several features of the radiation from a particular astronomical object. This requires the use of special instruments, suitable for both observing various types of astronomical objects and measuring various features of their radiation. The principal astronomical instrument is the telescope, together with the ancillary instruments mounted on it for particular purposes. The purpose of the telescopeis to provide, on an appropriate scale, the brightest possible image of the part of the sky under study.

Section 7   Telescopes

Inasmuch as the purpose of the telescope is to produce an image of the part of the sky under investigation, it must be an instrument which is capable of collecting a parallel beam of radiation from the largest possible area and focusing it at one point to produce a real image of the luminous object. The reflection and refraction of light are utilized to achieve this purpose.

In reflection, a ray of light changes its direction upon encountering a reflecting surface (mirror) so that the angle α between the incident ray and the normal to the mirror surface at the point of incidence (angle of incidence) is equal to the angle β between the reflected ray and that normal (angle of reflection). The incident and reflected rays and the normal to the surface of the mirror lie in one plane (Cf. Fig. 1-14).

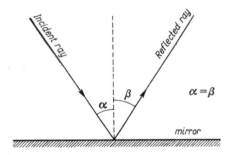

Figure 1-14. Reflection of light ray from a mirror.

Of course, if a parallel beam of the ray is incident on a plane mirror, the beam remains parallel after reflection. Conversely, if the surface of the mirror is not plane, a beam of nonparallel rays is obtained when a parallel beam is reflected. This property enables light radiation to be focused by choosing an appropriate shape of mirror. To focus a parallel beam of light at one point the mirror should be given the shape of a paraboloid of revolution with its axis parallel to the direction of the radiation (Cf. Fig. 1-15). Even with a paraboloidal mirror, however, a parallel beam of rays whose direction does not coincide with that of the optical axis of the mirror will not be focused at one point after reflection and images lying beyond the optical axis will, therefore, be blurred.

In a telescope with a mirror of this kind the image of an object is produced in front of the mirror. If measuring instruments used to study the

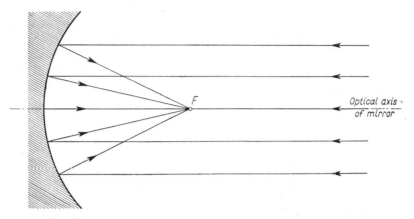

Figure 1-15. Reflection of parallel beam of light from a paraboloidal mirror. The rays converge at the focal point F of the mirror.

resultant image were installed at this spot, they would obscure a considerable part of the mirror and thus reduce the amount of radiation received. Moreover, it would be inconvenient to work with instruments inside the telescope housing. For that reason devices are used to direct the beam of light reflected from the mirror to a point outside the tube of the telescope: either to the side or behind the main mirror.

The first of these imaging devices was introduced by Newton who mounted a small flat mirror before the focus at an angle of 45° to the optical axis of the telescope (Cf. Fig. 1-16). In this case, the focus is at

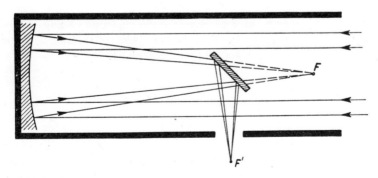

Figure 1-16. A Newtonian telescope.

the side of the telescope, where the measuring instruments are set up. With this arrangement the focal length (the distance from the focus to the mirror) is not altered.

In another arrangement a small hole is provided in the centre of the objective mirror so as to let through a beam of light reflected from a smaller, convex hyperboloidal mirror mounted before the focus (Cf. Fig. 1-17). This arrangement was introduced by Cassegrain. In the Cassegrain telescope measuring instruments are installed behind the principal mirror. In this case the focal length of the telescope is increased by the addition of the hyperboloidal mirror.

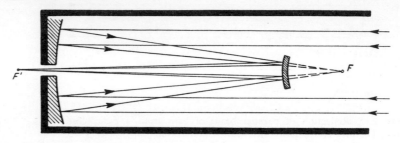

Figure 1-17. A Cassegrain telescope.

Telescopes utilizing mirrors to focus the beam of light are reflecting telescopes or reflectors. Other kinds of telescopes—refractors—make use of refraction of light to focus the beam of light. In refraction, a ray of light is bent at the interface separating two media. The angle between the incident ray and the normal to the interface at the point of incidence (angle of incidence i_1) and the angle between the refracted ray and that normal (angle of refraction i_2) obey the relation

$$\frac{\sin i_1}{\sin i_2} = \frac{n_2}{n_1},$$
(1-30)

where n_1 and n_2 are the indices of refraction in front of and behind the refracting surface (Fig. 1-18). The incident and refracted rays and the normal to the refracting surface all lie in one plane.

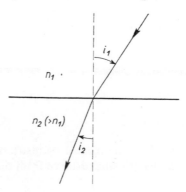

Figure 1-18. Refraction of a light ray.

This phenomenon is utilized to focus a parallel beam of light by the use of specially shaped lenses made of glass with an appropriate index of refraction. However, inasmuch as the index of refraction in glass depends on the wavelength of the incident radiation, rays of different colours focus at different points (Fig. 1-19). This defect of optical instruments is called

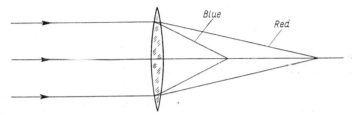

Figure 1-19. Chromatic aberration.

chromatic or colour aberration. Another major defect is that light rays focus at different points along the optical axis, depending on how far off the axis they were when passing through the lens (Fig. 1-20). This is known as spherical aberration. There is also considerable loss of light in large lenses. As a result refractors are now used less frequently than reflectors in astrophysical investigations.

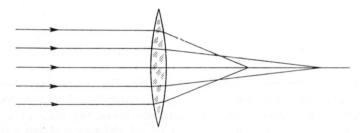

Figure 1-20. Spherical aberration.

To eliminate these aberrations, or at least to reduce them substantially, refractors are provided with objectives consisting of systems of lenses made of various types of glass with carefully chosen refractive indices and surface shapes. In practice, we never completely eliminate chromatic aberration for all wavelengths and we thus select a suitable system of lenses which reduce aberrations to a minimum in the spectral interval in which we wish to carry out observations.

Upon passing through the objective, radiation from astronomical objects forms an inverted real image at a distance equal to the focal length of that objective. This image may be recorded, e.g. on a photographic plate placed there. Beyond the focal length of the objective, visual telescopes have an ocular which magnifies the image produced by the objective. Of course, the objective should also be free of aberration and for that reason it, too, consists of a system of several lenses. The diagram of a visual refractor is shown in Fig. 1-21.

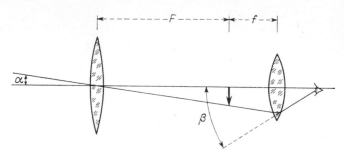

Figure 1-21. Diagram of a visual refractor.

Just as reflectors, refractors also have an aberration called coma such that images formed off the optical axis of telescope are distorted. This aberration grows with the distance from the optimal axis and, therefore, puts an upper limit on the radius of the region in which images are of adequate quality. The optical system of any telescope which we should like to use for simultaneous observations of a large part of the sky should be free of off-axis aberrations. This condition is met by a mirror whose surface composes part of the surface of a sphere. Indeed, if use is made of a spherical mirror, which means a mirror having no preferred axis, no direction will be privileged. A telescope of this kind, just as all reflector telescopes, will have no chromatic aberration. This mirror will, however, display spherical aberration since only the paraboloidal mirror does not suffer from this defect. Hence, a thin glass correcting plate of a shape chosen so as to compensate for the spherical aberration of the mirror is mounted in front of the mirror, at the centre of curvature of the latter. A telescope with such an optical system is called a Schmidt camera, after the man who invented it (Fig. 1-22). Such cameras are used extensively in astronomy to photograph large areas of the sky, whereas Cassegrain telescopes are employed to study individual objects.

A parallel beam of rays is never focused at one point even if all aberrations are eliminated in the telescope. This is due to diffraction of light. In telescopes this phenomenon consists in the interference of rays of light— from the same beam—arriving from various points of the objective (lens or mirror). Since the distances between various points of the objective and various points of the focal plane are not the same, rays arriving at a given point in the focal plane from various points of the objective will have

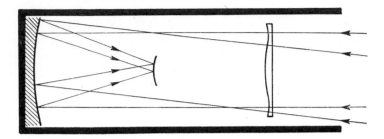

Figure 1-22. Diagram of a Schmidt camera.

travelled different paths and will thus be out of phase with each other. Consequently (as we known from Sec. 2), these rays will interfere. We shall observe constructive interference at some points of the focal plane and destructive interference at others. As a result the bright image of the object will be surrounded by a series of alternately bright and dark diffraction rings decreasing in brightness with distance from the centre. The radii of these rings depend on the wavelength λ of the light and on the diameter d of the telescope objective. The radius ϱ of the first dark diffraction ring (thus at the same time the radius of the central image) is given by the formula

$$\varrho = 1.22 \frac{\lambda}{d}, \tag{1-31}$$

where ϱ is in radians, and λ and d are in the same units of length. Two objects with an angular separation of less than ϱ form images which overlap considerably and these images cannot be resolved by the given telescope. Thus the value ϱ defines the resolving power of the telescope. In the region of visible radiation

$$\varrho \approx \frac{14''}{d}, \tag{1-32}$$

where ϱ is in seconds of arc, and d in cm. The effective resolving power of a telescope is affected adversely, of course, by the existence of aberrations and poor atmospheric conditions. Atmospheric distortion is particularly noticeable in large telescopes where the radii of diffraction rings are small.

Two point objects whose directions differ by an angle α (in radians) yield in the focal plane of the telescope images separated by

$$l = \alpha f, \tag{1-33}$$

where f is the focal length of the telescope (Fig. 1-23). Thus, the area A of the image of an extended object (large enough for the distorting influence

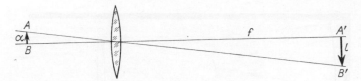

Figure 1-23. Distance of images of two objects A and B.

of diffraction to be neglected) is proportional to the solid angle Ω at which this object is seen and the square of the focal length, i.e.

$$A = \Omega f^2. \qquad (1\text{-}34)$$

Since the amount of energy reaching the telescope per unit time is proportional to the objective diameter squared d^2, the surface brightness of the image of an extended object is proportional to d^2/f^2. The quantity d/f is called the focal ratio or "speed" of the telescope. The speed does not, however, determine the surface brightness of the images of point objects (such as stars) since the diameters of these images depend on the extent of the diffraction and aberration in the telescope.

Such properties as the focal length, diameter of the objective, size of the field of observation, and transmissivity of particular parts of the spectrum predispose various types of telescopes to particular types of astronomical observations. In choosing a telescope, one must bear in mind what kind of objects are to be observed and what features of their radiation are to be investigated.

Mountings which enable telescopes to be set in a desired direction and moved to follow the rotation of the celestial sphere are placed on massive foundations which ensure stability. The building which houses a telescope is covered with a movable roof, usually a dome with a shuttered slot.

Section 8   Recording the Image

The area of the sky under study is imaged in the focal plane of the telescope, and this image can be studied directly or from a record of it. The resultant recorded image can be stored, reproduced, transmitted, and then measured under more convenient conditions. Depending on the technique employed, there are two main types of record: chemical and electromagnetic.

Chemical records are made by using a photographic plate. This usually consists of a glass plate coated with a light-sensitive emulsion consisting of a suspension of a silver salt in gelatine. After exposure, the photographic plate is processed in the laboratory to develop and fix the image. The image so recorded is a negative of the observed field, i.e. bright objects such as stars yield dark images. The blackening of the plate, however, is a function not only of the illumination of the source but also of the exposure time.

By choosing a sufficiently long exposure we can obtain images of fainter and fainter objects. The maximum exposure time, however, is limited since it is not possible to maintain exactly the same conditions of exposure over a long period of time. Variations in the ambient temperature cause changes in the plate sensitivity, and affect the optics of the instrument; moreover, the optical properties of the atmosphere also vary. However, as the exposure time is extended there is an increase in the overall blackening of the plate owing to the night sky light.

It is the aim of the observer that the image produced on the plate be a faithful representation of the part of the sky under study. The point is not only that the position of the images on the plate correspond to that of the observed objects in the sky but also that the ratios of the blackenings of images on the plate be the simplest possible, single-valued function of the ratio of the intensities of radiation received. This is associated with the exposure time (depending on the brightness of the observed objects), the type of telescope, and the quality of photographic plate. To this end we must know how the photographic plate reacts to radiation incident on it or, in other words, we must know how the blackening of the plate is related to the amount of light to which it is exposed. This relationship is known as the characteristic of the plate (Fig. 1-24). The opaqueness of the

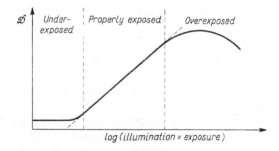

Figure 1-24. Characteristic of a photographic plate.

plate can be used as a measure of its blackening. If we direct a luminous flux of intensity I_0 at a given point on a developed plate, light of a reduced intensity I (depending on the degree of blackening) will be transmitted by that point on the plate. The value

$$\mathscr{D} = \log \frac{I_0}{I} \qquad (1\text{-}35)$$

can be treated as a measure of blackening; this is plotted in Fig. 1-24. The shape of the plate characteristic shows that too brief as well as too long exposure times are undesirable. For proper exposure of the plate the exposure time must be chosen so that the images of the objects studied lie on the rectilinear section of the characteristic curve. Only then can we easily and uniquely determine the ratios of illuminations. It should be noted, however, that each photographic plate has a different characteristic since identical conditions cannot be maintained during production, storage, and development of the plate. The characteristic must, therefore, be determined separately for each plate.

It is important to have a plate with a characteristic curve which is linear over a large interval. This problem has been solved in recent years by the use of electron-optical image converters. These devices operate on the principle of the photoelectric effect. In this process light falling on a metal surface knocks electrons out of that surface, the number of electrons knocked out being proportional to the intensity of the incident light while their energy is linearly dependent on the frequency of the radiation. In an electron-optical image converter the image of the object being observed is projected onto the cathode which emits a beam of electrons. This beam passes through an appropriate arrangement of electromagnetic lenses which direct it at an electron-sensitive plate such that every electron incident on it causes one grain of the emulsion to be blackened. It is thus seen that when image converters are used, the plate characteristic curve becomes linear over a very broad range: the number of blackened grains is proportional to the number of electrons, and this in turn is proportional to the illumination. A second advantage provided by the use of image converters is an increase in the sensitivity of the plate. The number of electrons knocked out of the cathode by the given number of photons is much greater than the number of emulsion grains blackened when the same number of photons is directly incident on the plate. This makes it possible to photograph faint objects which would not be observable without the aid of image converters.

Image converters of the type described above, however, are tedious to use because a high vacuum has to be maintained in them. A high vacuum is necessary in order to ensure rectilinear propagation of electrons which would otherwise be scattered by molecules of air. In converters in which electrons are projected directly onto a plate, the vacuum is "destroyed" after each observation when the plate is replaced by a new one. For this reason, another arrangement is employed: the electrons are incident on a fluorescent screen producing an image of the observed object. This image can then be photographed. Here, the cathode, system of lenses, and fluorescent screen are inside a housing which ensures a vacuum. The photographic plate is outside the housing and its replacement does not require any additional procedures. Some of the quality of the images obtained is, however, lost in such converters.

In the foregoing methods the image is recorded by being formed on a photographic plate, either directly or by means of an electron image converter. However, when a converter is used the image may be recorded on magnetic tape rather than a photographic plate. In many cases a television camera is used as an image converter and the image can be transmitted over long distances; the instrument with which we perform the observations may be far from the place where the image is recorded. This technique is highly important for observations carried out beyond the atmosphere by means of artificial satellites and space vehicles.

Section 9   Photometry

One of the most frequent activities of an observer is to measure the intensity of radiation arriving from an astronomical object under study. The branch of astronomy devoted to these measurements is called photometry. Direct photometric measurements may be performed on the image formed by a telescope. If the image is first recorded on a photographic plate, we speak of photographic photometry.

In the preceding section, the value of $\mathscr{D}$ defined by Eq. (1-35) was

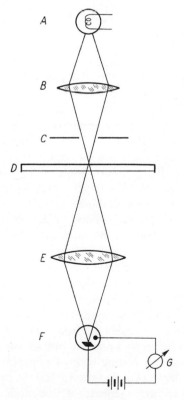

Figure 1-25. A photometer for measuring plate blackening.

taken as a measure of the blackening of the plate. The definition of $\mathscr{D}$ as the logarithm of the ratio of intensities of incident light and light transmitted by a given spot on the plate prescribes the method of using a photometer. In a photometer for measuring photographic plates (Fig. 1-25), a beam of light from source A is directed by means of objective B at the star image to be measured on plate D. This beam passes through the diaphragm C which limits the illumination field on the plate. After traversing the plate, the beam is focused onto the cathode of the photocell F by the objective lens E. The photographic plate is arranged so that the stellar image is in the centre of the illuminated field and the current i_1 in the circuit of G is measured. The plate is then placed so that the light passes through the blackened places on it and the current i_2 is noted. Since the current is proportional to the illumination of the photocathode, we may write

$$\mathscr{D} = \log \frac{i_2}{i_1}. \tag{1-36}$$

Once the value of $\mathscr{D}$ has been measured in this way for a number of stars, the characteristic curve of the given plate can be used to determine the ratios of the illumination of the radiation from these stars. If the brightness of some of these stars is known, this method permits direct determination of the illumination due to the observed radiation. The accuracy of this method is conditional first and foremost upon the quality of the images on the plate and is no better than 2%. However, its principal advantage is that material for measuring the brightness of a large number of stars can be obtained on one plate during a single observation.

Much more accurate results are provided by the methods of photoelectric photometry. In this case, no image is recorded on a photographic plate but instead a beam of light from a star is collected by a telescope and directed straight at a photocathode. Usually, instead of the image of the star itself, the image of the telescope objective illuminated by the light of that star is projected onto the photocathode by means of an auxiliary lens. This eliminates the undesirable influence of nonuniform sensitivity at various places on the photocathode surface; this influence would make itself felt if an almost point image were to move over that surface. The radiation of other stars and the background of the sky is removed by inserting a diaphragm of suitable diameter in the path of the beam of light. Photomultipliers are used in photoelectric photometers in order to amplify the beam of electrons knocked out of the photocathode by the stellar radiation. A diagram of one type of photomultiplier used is shown in Fig. 1-26 as an example. The main elements of this photomultiplier are a photocathode and an arrangement of 9 dynodes and an anode. The potential difference between the cathode and anode is about 100 volts,

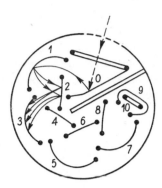

Figure 1-26. Diagram of a 1P21 photomultiplier.

and between two consecutive dynodes, 100 volts. Stellar light incident on
the cathode knocks out a stream of electrons which is focused onto the
first dynode. In the best present-day photomultipliers approximately one in
every three photons knocks an electron out of the cathode. Each electron
incident on a dynode causes secondary emission of several electrons (three
or four in the case of the 1P21 photomultiplier). The now reinforced beam
of electrons is accelerated to the second dynode, and from there on to the
next, and so on. The multiplying effect is repeated at each dynode by
secondary emission. Thus, the original beam of electrons is subjected to
considerable multiplication, of the order of 10^6 in 1P21 photomultipliers.
The photomultiplier current is passed through an amplifier and then usually
recorded by means of a recorder.

Considerable advances were achieved with the introduction of photon
counters. Photons striking a photomultiplier cathode cause only single
electrons to be knocked out. A stream of electrons initiated in the multi-
plier by these electrons yields a pulse of current at the output. These pulses
are counted and the number of pulses per second is proportional to the
illumination of the photocathode with radiation from a star.

Each set of instruments used in photometry displays a different sensitivity in the various colours. Thus, measurements of the brightness of astronomical objects by means of different instruments can not be compared
directly. In speaking of the brightness of some object, we always assume
the brightness of that object in some particular part of the spectrum. If
a given set of instruments is to be used to measure the brightness of stars
in a particular colour, it is necessary to employ filters which transmit only
radiation of that colour. However, it must be borne in mind that the results
depend not only on the filters used but also on the entire set of instruments:
telescope, filters, and type of photomultiplier or photographic plate.

Polarization of stellar light is measured with polarimeters—instruments which are similar to photoelectric photometers as far as principle of operation is concerned. Placement of a polarizer in front of the photomultiplier photocathode makes polarimeters suitable for measurements of polarization. This polarizer can be rotated about the optical axis of the instrument. Measurements with the polarizer in several positions determine both the degree and direction of the polarization.

Section 10   Spectroscopy

The use of filters in photometric observations enables us to study the intensity of stellar radiation in individual colours. More precise information about the spectral distribution, however, is provided by spectrographs. The purpose of spectrographs is to spread the light of stars so that radiation at each wavelength focuses a different place in the focal plane. This is accomplished by exploiting either the wavelength-dependence of the index of refraction or the phenomenon of diffraction. Light is broken up in a prism (Fig. 1-27) in the first case, and on a diffraction grating in the second.

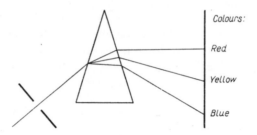

Figure 1-27. Light spread by a prism.

A diffraction grating may consist of a number of parallel equidistant slits of identical width, separated by partitions which are opaque to light. Most frequently, however, diffraction gratings are made on the surfaces of mirrors. In this case, the diffraction grating consists of a number of parallel equidistant rulings on the mirror. A parallel beam of radiation passing through (or reflected from) a grating undergoes diffraction, that is, waves arriving from different slits (rulings) interfere to produce a number of images called diffraction images. With the exception of the zero-order image, these images are spectra of the incident radiation (Fig. 1-28). If the rulings on the mirror are of a suitable profile, about 70 per cent of the light can be concentrated in a given spectrum.

In general, a spectrograph consists of: a collimator (a lens which forms a parallel beam of light), a prism or diffraction grating, and a lens to focus the dispersed beam of light. However, not all of these components are found in all spectrographs used in astronomy.

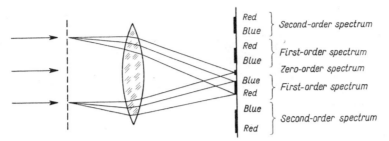

Figure 1-28. Formation of diffraction patterns.

One of the simplest types of instruments for obtaining a spectrum is the objective prism. Since parallel beams of stellar radiation fall on the objective of a telescope, no collimator is required if a prism is placed in front of the objective of the telescope (best of all, a Schmidt camera). The beam is broken up in the prism (or suitable system of prisms) and then falls on the objective of the telescope whose entire optical system serves only to focus the spectrum image in the focal plane (Fig. 1-29). Spectra of all stars in

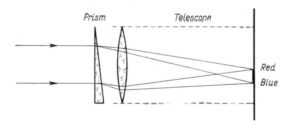

Figure 1-29. An objective prism.

the field of observation are formed there. A photographic plate put in the focal plane of the telescope records simultaneously the spectral images of many stars (Plate 2). The ability to collect a considerable number of spectra during a single observation is the principal attribute of the objective prism. It does, however, have a number of disadvantages in comparison to other spectrographs. The main disadvantages of spectra obtained by means of an objective prism include: low dispersion (i.e. the length of the spectral interval, expressed in units of wavelength, is large compared to the length of the image of that interval), blurring of the spectrum by vibrations during exposure of the plate, errors in the telescope motion, and partial superposition of the spectra of neighbouring stars.

Another type of spectrograph is the slit spectrograph, which is shown schematically in Fig. 1-30. In this type of instrument, the light passes through a slit placed in the focal plane of the telescope so that an observed

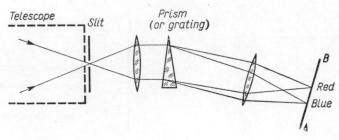

Figure 1-30. Diagram of a slit spectograph.

star is imaged on the slit. A collimator turns the beam of light from the slit into a parallel beam which passes through a prism or is reflected from a diffraction grating, and is then broken up into a number of monochromatic beams. When focused by a special objective, each of the monochromatic beams forms an image of the slit at a different place on the plate, depending on the wavelength. In a spectrum so obtained the distribution of intensities can also be measured by a photomultiplier moving along the straight line AB in Fig. 1-30 or, again, electron-optical image converters may be used instead of a photographic plate.

To avoid losses of stellar light at the spectrograph slit, relatively wide slits of no less than 0.1 mm are usually used. However, the slit images formed should be reduced considerably in size so that the spectrum pro-

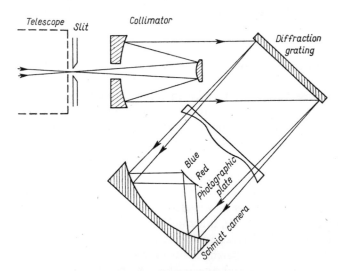

Figure 1-31. A slit spectrograph with diffraction grating, an inverted Cassegrain telescope as collimator, and a Schmidt camera as focusing objective.

duced on the photographic plate is sharp. This is achieved when the focal ratio (or speed) of the objective focusing the dispersed beam of light is higher than that of the spectrograph collimator. For this reason, an inverted Cassegrain (Fig. 1-31) with the same speed as the main telescope usually serves as the collimator in astronomical slit spectrographs while a Schmidt camera of high speed (sometimes as much as 1:0.5) serves as the focusing objective.

One of the advantages of the slit spectrograph is that comparison spectra can be obtained. The stellar image occupies only part of the slit area. If the rest of the slit is illuminated with comparison radiation having a known distribution of spectral lines (Fig. 1-32), the plate will have the comparison

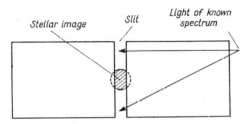

Figure 1-32. A stellar image in a slit. The rest of the slit can be illuminated with radiation with known distribution of spectral lines.

spectrum next to the stellar spectrum (Plate 3). This considerably facilitates identification of lines and bands in the stellar spectrum and also enables their position to be measured. The slit spectrograph thus is particularly suited for measuring the radial velocities of stars. Another advantage of the slit spectrograph over the objective prism is that stellar spectra can be obtained with high dispersions, up to as much as 2 Å/mm, while the maximum dispersion of the objective prism is about 100 Å/mm.

Section 11   Heliophysical Instruments

Heliophysical instruments are set apart from other instruments employed in astronomy because observations of the Sun are made under quite different conditions. One of the principal difficulties in the observation of stars is that only a small amount of radiation is received. This limits the accuracy of the results obtained in many cases. These difficulties do not attend the study of the Sun, however. The great surface brightness of the solar disk makes it possible for us to get considerable magnifications of portions of the solar surface and to study their structure. It also enables high-dispersion spectra to be obtained.

Large magnifications, however, require the use of telescopes with very long focal length. Thus, in heliophysical observations we must resort to a construction quite different from those of telescopes employed to observe the stars. In solar observations it becomes vital to eliminate the influence of atmospheric turbulence (which is much more pronounced in the day than at night) inasmuch as it causes the images to be blurred and to vibrate in the focal plane of the telescope. Consequently, the tower telescope which has its objective on a tower several tens of metres above the ground is frequently used. It is placed at a height sufficient for atmospheric turbulence to be much reduced. Measuring instruments are installed in an appropriate well beneath the tower, where a constant temperature is maintained (Fig. 1-33). Since tower telescopes are immobile (this is necessary in view

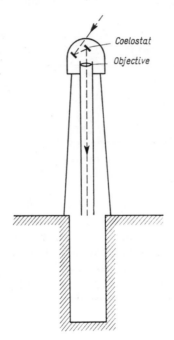

Figure 1-33. Sketch of a tower telescope.

of the long focal length), auxiliary devices must be used to bring to the objective radiation from the Sun as it moves across the sky. An example of such a device, called a coelostat, is shown in Fig. 1-34. Mirror *1* rotates about axis *AB* to follow the Sun (but at half the velocity) so that solar rays are reflected from it on to mirror *2*. The purpose of mirror *2* is to reflect incident radiation downwards, on to the objective of the telescope.

Since the solar disk is of considerable angular dimensions, the spectrum of the Sun can be studied only by using slit spectrographs. With slits, however, the spectrum of only a narrow strip of the solar disk is obtained

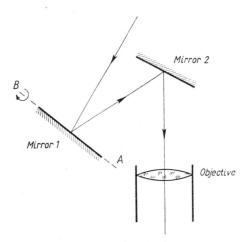

Figure 1-34. Sketch of a coelostat.

on a photographic plate during a single observation. In many cases the observer is interested in getting an image of the entire Sun in monochromatic light, i.e. in one specific spectral line. This enables him to study how the constituent absorbing or emitting that line is distributed in the solar atmosphere. Such monochromatic images of the Sun are obtained with the spectroheliograph. This instrument (Fig. 1-35) is similar in construction to slit spectrographs. A major difference is that an additional slit in front of the photographic plate cuts out radiation of the desired wavelength, producing a monochromatic image of one strip of the Sun. Both slits are

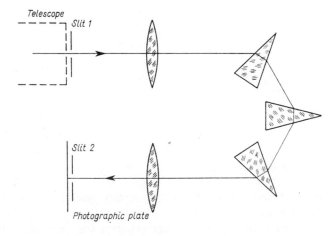

Figure 1-35. Diagram of a spectroheliograph.

then moved vertically in the same direction together with the set of prisms (Fig. 1-35) so that images of successive strips of the Sun are formed at slit *1*. Since slit *2* moves in front of the photographic plate, monochromatic images of successive strips of the solar disk are formed next to each other. The resultant image of the Sun is called a spectroheliogram (Cf. Plate 17).

The possibility of obtaining large dispersions of the solar spectrum also permits accurate measurements of the solar magnetic field. In this case use is made of the Zeeman effect. The spectral lines of radiation from gases in a magnetic field are split into several components. In the direction perpendicular to the magnetic field, lines are split into three linearly polarized components: the outer components are polarized normal to the magnetic field, while the middle components are parallel to it. On the other hand, if observations are made from a direction parallel to the magnetic field, the spectral line is seen to be split into two components circularly polarized in opposite directions. The separation of the components depends on the intensity of the magnetic field in which the radiating gas happens to be. Thus, measurement of this separation for the components of any line in radiation from a particular place on the solar disk provides information about the intensity of the magnetic field existing there. The difficulty is that in areas beyond sunspots, the magnetic field is so weak that the separation of components in much less than their width. In ordinary spectrophotometric observations, the two components will be superposed on each other, thus preventing measurement of the distance between them. This difficulty has been overcome by using the solar magnetograph (Fig. 1-36).

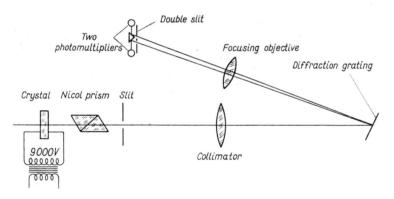

Figure 1-36. Diagram of a solar magnetograph.

The solar magnetograph contains a polarizer placed in front of a slit spectrograph; in brief intervals of time this polarizer transmits radiation alternately from each of the two components of the split line, circularly polarized in opposite directions. This radiation comes out of the spectrograph through two slits (Fig. 1-37) to fall on two photomultipliers beyond them. The polarizer used in the magnetograph consists of a crystal plate under high voltage and a Nicol prism. This arrangement transmits circularly polarized radiation in one direction, depending on the sign of the potential

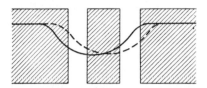

Figure 1-37. The double slit of a solar magnetograph illuminated with light from the components of a split line. The solid and dashed lines represent the distribution of radiation intensity in the line components.

on the crystal plate. When the sign of the potential on the crystal plate is changed rapidly (in practice, 120 Hz), the photocathodes of the multipliers are illuminated alternately by one component and the other (Fig. 1-37). Since the positions of the two components differ slightly from each other, variations in the photocathode illumination ensue. The greater the separation of the components, the more pronounced are these variations. The multipliers are incorporated into a circuit so that the difference in the illuminations of the two photocathodes is recorded. Consequently, the 120-Hz changes in the current in the circuit are due only to the fact that the components of the line are in different positions in the spectrum: they do not depend on slow variations of illumination owing to changes in extinction in the terrestrial atmosphere, for example. Measurements of many points on the solar disk provide a means for reproducing the topography of the solar magnetic field at a given time (Plate 4). Magnetic fields of 0.5 gauss on the Sun can be detected with a magnetograph; the Zeeman splitting which corresponds to this field intensity is merely about 10^{-5} Å.

The Zeeman effect is also utilized to study the magnetic fields of stars. Inasmuch as stars are much dimmer, we cannot use spectrographs of very high dispersing power nor can we employ a magnetograph of the type described above. Consequently, instruments in service at present are capable of detecting only strong stellar magnetic fields which yield considerable separation of the components of the line undergoing Zeeman splitting.

Section 12 Radioastronomical Instruments

The advances made in radio engineering, which were particularly rapid after World War II, inaugurated a new field in astronomy: the study of the radio-frequency emission from astronomical objects. A number of devices have been built to pick up this radiation and the principal types will be discussed in this section. An antenna and a receiver are the main components of these devices.

The simplest antenna is a half-wave dipole which consists of two rods arranged in a straight line and connected to a receiver by wires. The total length of the dipole equals half the wavelength of the radiation being measured. When the dipole length is so chosen, the oscillations of the electric vector of radiation and the oscillations of the electric charges in the dipole enter into resonance. Since these oscillations take place in a plane perpendicular to the propagation direction of the wave, the dipole exhibits greatest sensitivity to radiation arriving from directions perpendicular to it but does not record radiation incident along the dipole axis (Fig. 1-38). As indicated by Fig. 1-38b, a dipole antenna picks up

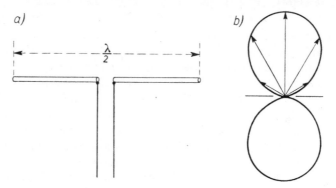

Figure 1-38. A half-wave dipole: a) appearance; b) the directional characteristic (receiving pattern) of the dipole (the length of the vectors shown is proportional to the ratio of the intensity of the current induced by radiation arriving from a given direction to the intensity of that radiation). To obtain the spatial pattern, the figure shown in (b) should be rotated about the dipole axis.

radiation from a large area of the sky and, therefore, cannot be used to pinpoint exactly the location of the source of radio emission under study.

Radiotelescopes are used in order to ensure that the radio waves received come from a particular direction. A dipole or some other type of antenna is placed at the focus of a paraboloidal metal surface in radiotelescopes. Radio wavelength emission from the direction of the paraboloid axis is focused on the dipole after reflection from the paraboloidal surface. At the same time, this surface shields the dipole from radiation from other parts of the sky. The resolving power of radiotelescopes (as in the case of optical telescopes) is determined by the size of the diffraction image:

$$\varrho = 1.22\lambda/d \qquad (1\text{-}31)$$

(Cf. p. 19). Since the radius of the diffraction image is proportional to the wavelength, the diameter of the radiotelescope must be large if the resolving power is to be satisfactory. However, even large radiotelescopes do not have a high resolving power. In the case of a radiotelescope 100 metres in diameter, for example, the radius of the diffraction image for wavelengths of 1 metre is 42' and the position of a radiating object in the sky can be determined only to this accuracy. Paraboloidal reflectors increase the sensitivity of the antenna since the amount of energy reaching it per unit time is proportional to the square of the reflector diameter. The reflecting surface most frequently consists of a lattice of metal rods. Such a lattice acts as a reflector for waves with wavelengths at least several times the diameter of the lattice meshes. Use of a lattice instead of a solid metal surface reduces the weight of the entire structure and thus considerably facilitates assembly and operation of the radiotelescope.

Another arrangement which enhances the directivity of the antenna employs an array of dipoles. A pair of dipoles separated by $\lambda/2$ and connected as shown in Fig. 1-39a does not pick up radiation from directions

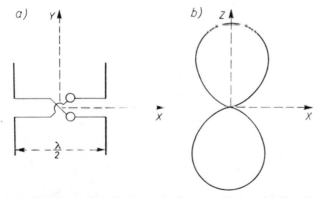

Figure 1-39. A pair of crossed dipoles: a) diagram; b) the directional characteristic of the system (to obtain the spatial pattern, the figure shown in (b) should be rotated about the Z axis).

in the plane of the system. Indeed, radiation arriving from the X direction sets up in both dipoles oscillations which are out of phase with each other by 180°. Since the dipoles are crossed, these oscillations cancel out at the input to the receiver. Radiation from the Y direction, parallel to the axes of both dipoles, does not induce any oscillations at all in the dipoles. Only radiation from directions with a nonvanishing Z component— perpendicular to the plane of the array—sets up oscillations in phase with each other in both dipoles and this radiation is recorded by the receiver. The directional characteristic or receiving pattern of such an arrangement is shown in Fig. 39b. A pair of crossed dipoles receives radiation from a much smaller area of the sky than does a single dipole. Nevertheless, this area is still of considerable size since it constitutes about 30 per cent of the entire sky. For better directivity, collinear arrays of many dipoles arranged in series in one plane are used. The receiving angle of such antennae is inversely proportional to their size.

In the case of paraboloidal and collinear-array radiotelescopes alike, the resolving power increases with the dimensions. However, an antenna with a sufficiently small receiving angle, especially for longer waves (of several metres) would be several hundred metres in size. This entails many constructional and operational difficulties. Consequently, the problem of further reducing the receiving angle is solved in a different way. Interference of waves is exploited for this purpose and instruments operating on this principle are called interferometers. The simplest interferometer is an array of two dipoles at a considerable distance D from each other (Fig. 1-40). Let us consider radiation which is incident (in the plane of

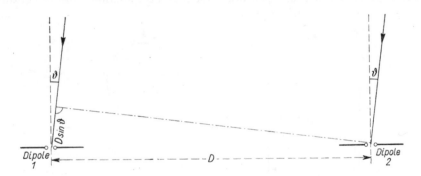

Figure 1-40. The principle of the interferometer.

the drawing) upon an interferometer at an angle ϑ. The path this radiation traverses to dipole 1 is $D\sin\vartheta$ longer than that to dipole 2. Consequently, the radio waves received simultaneously by the two dipoles are displaced in wavelength with respect to each other by $D\sin\vartheta$. If this displacement is a multiple of the wavelength, that is if

$$D\sin\vartheta = n\lambda \quad (n = 0, \pm1, \pm2, ...) \tag{1-37}$$

the signal is amplified. Thus the receiver will record radiation arriving from directions for which

$$\sin\vartheta = n\lambda/D \quad (n = 0, \pm1, \pm2, ...). \tag{1-38}$$

If, on the other hand, radiation is received from directions for which

$$\sin\vartheta = (n+\tfrac{1}{2})\lambda/D \quad (n = 0, \pm1, \pm2, ...) \tag{1-39}$$

the oscillations in the two dipoles are out of phase by 180° and cancel at the receiver input. The directional pattern of an interferometer (Cf. Fig. 1-41a) thus consists of a number of lobes indicating the directions from which the interferometer receives radiation. The width of these

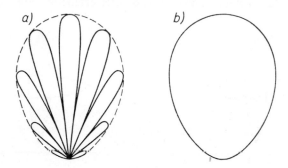

Figure 1-41. The directional characteristic of an interferometer: a) in the plane of the interferometer; b) in a plane perpendicular to its axis.

lobes [Cf. Eq. (1-39)] for a given wavelength is inversely proportional to the distance D between dipoles. However, the resolving power of the interferometer in a plane perpendicular to its axis is low, just as for a single dipole (Cf. Fig. 1-41b). Interferometers are also used with arrays of dipoles or reflectors set up in series. The principal lobe of the receiving pattern is then lengthened considerably while the adjoining ones are almost completely suppressed.

In order to attain the necessary high resolving power in studies of radio sources of very small angular size, simultaneous measurements are made with two (or more) radio telescopes a large distance apart, perhaps even on different continents. In this case the base of the interferometric system amounts to thousands of kilometres; the resolving power of the system in centimetre waves is of the order of several ten-thousandths of a second of arc. Inasmuch as they are so far apart, the radio telescopes composing such an interferometer are not connected directly to a receiver. Instead, the phases of the radiation received from the radio sources are recorded independently but simultaneously on magnetic tapes which also record signals from two previously synchronized atomic clocks. Comparison of the two tapes by means of computers yields all the information obtainable from conventional interferometers but the resolving power is increased radically.

Since ordinary interferometers have a low resolving power in directions perpendicular to their axes, interferometer systems with mutually perpendicular axes are used. The Mills cross is an example of such an instrument. It consists of two crossed interferometers, each of which receives radiation from a strip of the sky perpendicular to its axis. Since the axes of the two interferometers are at right angles to each other, the two strips of the sky will intersect at a right angle (Fig. 1-42). Radiation arriving from the central area (cross-hatched in Fig. 1-42a) will be received by both interferometers. Thus, if the interferometers are connected to

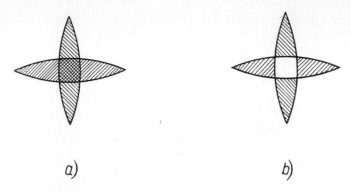

Figure 1-42. The principle of the Mills cross.

a receiver so that signals from them meet in phase at the receiver input, the sensitivity of the arrangement will be greater at the intersection of the two lobes than in the other parts of the sensitivity bands of the interferometers. If the interferometers are connected so that the signals from them meet at the receiver input in opposite phases, the system will be completely insensitive to radiation coming from the central area (Fig. 1-42b). The two interferometers are now rapidly switched so that the signals meet alternately in phase and out of phase by 180°. As a result, radiation arriving from the central area of the crossed lobes will produce at the receiver input an alternating signal with a frequency equal to the interferometer switching frequency. A receiver designed for this frequency will record only radiation in the central receiving beam. Consequently, the resolving power of the Mills cross is high, comparable with that of a paraboloidal radio telescope equal in diameter to the length of one of the component interferometers. A Mills cross with arms 3200 metres long operating at 10-metre waves has a resolving power of about 10′.

Electrical oscillations induced in the antenna are transmitted to the receiver. The antenna receives radiation over a wide range of frequencies, and the signals obtained from the antenna are very faint owing to the low intensity of the radio waves. Therefore, the purpose of the receiver is to select a signal at a particular frequency and, subsequently, to amplify it. The output from the receiver is an electric current with an intensity proportional to that of the radiation from the radio source.

Section 13 Observations Beyond the Atmosphere

Extension of the range of astronomical observations to the part of the spectrum lying beyond the atmospheric windows requires the placement of instruments outside the Earth's atmosphere. This has been made possible through the development of rocketry. Instruments installed in rockets, artificial satellites, and space vehicles can carry out measurements outside the terrestrial atmosphere and in interplanetary space, or can even be put on the surface of other bodies of the solar system. Some of the principal tasks confronting this new branch of astronomy are: to study the shape of the Earth and the distribution of the mass in its interior, to provide meteorological data, to make observations of the upper atmosphere and the propagation of radio waves within it, to determine the topography of the Earth's magnetic field, to make measurements of cosmic radiation, to observe meteors and interplanetary matter, to gain knowledge about the surface of the Moon and planets, to measure the photon and corpuscular radiation emitted by the Sun, stars, and interplanetary matter, and to obtain a more accurate value for the astronomical unit.

The use of artificial satellites and space vehicles enables new observational techniques to be introduced into many branches of science (geodesy, meteorology, geophysics, astronomy, physics, biology, medicine). The study of the motion of satellites and space vehicles provides information about the geometry of the gravitational field and the magnitude of the resistance offered by the medium, and hence about the shape and distribution of mass inside the body orbited by the given satellite, as well as about how the atmosphere surrounding that body varies with altitude; at the same time, observations of the position of artificial satellites from several points on the Earth are utilized for geodetical purposes. Rocket- and satellite-borne instruments (telescopes, spectrographs, and photometers sensitive to radiation which is absorbed in the atmosphere, magnetographs, particle counters, etc.) permit a direct examination of the upper atmosphere (the ionosphere, Van Allen belts) as well as of the topography of the terrestrial and interplanetary magnetic field. Moreover, they also enable scientists to make extra-atmospheric measurements of photon radiation (particularly in the infrared and the ultraviolet, and X-rays and gamma radiation) and corpuscular radiation from the Sun, stars, and clouds of interstellar material, as well as cosmic radiation. Research is also done in artificial satellites to determine how the conditions of space flight (above all, weightlessness, state of high acceleration force, and cosmic radiation) affect living organisms (plants, animals, and humans). Man-made satellites are used for radio and telecommunications (e.g. television relay stations) and for military purposes.

Data collected by instrumentation on board artificial satellites and space vehicles are transmitted by telemetry to ground receiving stations and, in the case of satellites and vehicles brought back down to Earth, are also recorded on data records, photographic plates, or magnetic tapes.

Manned space flights constitute a separate chapter. One should realize that we are witnesses to remarkable achievements symbolized by the names of Gagarin, Armstrong, Aldrin, and Collins, achievements paid for by the lives of Grissom, White, Chaffee, and Komarov. The efforts of many generations and nations have gone into the making of these achievements for which a comparison in the past can be found only in such stages in the development of life on Earth as when living organisms extended their sphere of existence beyond the watery habitat or when the protoplasts of the species today known as *homo sapiens* first assumed the upright position.

Chapter 2 The Motions of the Earth

Section 14 Rotation of the Earth

The conclusion that the Earth rotates on an axis passing through its interior may be drawn from observation of a number of phenomena occurring on the Earth's surface. One such proof is provided by the experiment performed by Foucault. He found that the plane of oscillation of a freely suspended pendulum undergoes rotation in respect to an observer on the surface of the Earth. This would not happen if the Earth did not rotate; in that case the motion of the pendulum would take place in a fixed plane. Other proofs of the existence of a Coriolis force due to the rotation of the Earth is given by the fact that falling bodies are deflected eastward from the vertical and that meridional winds are deflected (Cf. Sec. 23).

The apparent motion of the firmament is a reflection of the Earth's rotation. The concept of the celestial sphere is very useful in this context. The celestial sphere will be taken to mean a sphere of arbitrary radius with the observer at the centre. The position St_1 of an object on the celestial sphere will be identified with the point at which that sphere is pierced by the half-line from the observer O to the given object St (Fig. 2-1).

Since, in general, the distances to astronomical objects are much greater than the radius of the Earth we do not contribute any appreciable error

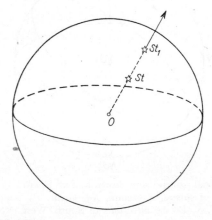

Figure 2-1. The celestial sphere.

by neglecting the size of the Earth and considering the observer to be at the centre of the Earth. With such procedure, however, we must bear in mind that the positions of nearby astronomical bodies (e.g. these within the solar system) on the celestial sphere will be different for observers at different points on the Earth. This fact is exploited in measurements of the distance to those bodies.

Because of the Earth's rotation, the positions of all astronomical objects in the sky change with time but the mutual configuration of these bodies is retained. We have the impression that the celestial sphere together with the objects on it, rotates on a specific diameter called the axis of the heavens (of course, it coincides in direction with the axis on which the Earth rotates). The axis of the heavens pierces the celestial sphere at two points called the celestial north and south poles (one of them—the north pole—can be seen only from the northern hemisphere of the Earth, and the other—the south pole—only from the southern hemisphere). A plane perpendicular to the axis of rotation and passing through the centre of the celestial sphere intersects that sphere in a great circle known as the celestial equator. This divides the celestial sphere into two hemispheres: the northern hemisphere which contains the celestial north pole and the southern hemisphere with the south pole.

The position of the equator and the poles in the sky depends on the geographical latitude φ at the point of observation. The angular distance of the celestial north pole from the zenith (the point at which the direction opposite to the force of gravity pierces the celestial sphere) is $90° - \varphi$.

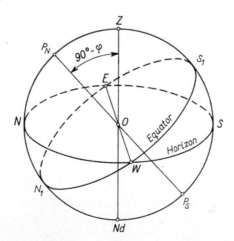

Figure 2-2. The celestial sphere with horizon and equator indicated. O—observer = centre of sphere, Z—zenith, Nd—nadir, P_N—north pole, P_S—south pole, S, W, N, E—the directions of South, West, North, and East.

The point diametrically opposite the zenith on the celestial sphere (invisible from the point of observation, of course) is called the nadir. A plane perpendicular to the direction of the force of gravity and passing through the point of observation intersects the celestial sphere along a great circle called the horizon. The position of the horizon and equator with respect to each other at a locality of geographical latitude φ is shown in Fig. 2-2. The great half-circle $P_N Z P_S$ is called the meridian. Point S at the intersection of the meridian and the horizon determines the direction of south. The opposite point on the celestial sphere, N, denotes the northerly direction and the points of intersection of the horizon and the equator, E and W, denote East and West, respectively. The point of intersection of the equator and the meridian is denoted by S_1 and the point on the celestial sphere opposite to it by N_1.

The descriptions presented above may be used to define two of the several systems of coordinates used in astronomy. These are: the horizon system of coordinates and the equator meridian system. Data characterizing these systems are listed in Table 2-1 (the notations and terms employed have been discussed in Sec. 5).

TABLE 2-1

Horizon and Equator-Meridian Systems

Principal Elements	Horizon	Equator-meridian
Reference plane P	horizon	equator
Reference direction $\mathbf{k}$	OS	OS_1
Name of angle U	azimuth: A	hour angle: t
Direction of increase of angle U	SWNE	$S_1 W N_1 E$
Range of angle U	0 to 360°	0 to 24^h
Name of angle V	altitude*: h	declination: δ
Range of angle V	−90 to +90°	−90 to +90°

* The zenith distance to the star, $z = 90° - h$, is frequently given instead of the altitude h.

The hour angle is measured (westward between the celestial meridian plane and the plane running across the poles and a star) in hours (1^h), minutes (1^m) and seconds (1^s). Since by definition an angle of 360° is equal to 24^h, then $1^h = 15°$, $1^m = 15'$, and $1^s = 15''$. The coordinates of star St in Fig. 2-3 are given in both systems mentioned above.

During the diurnal motion of the celestial sphere the stars move along celestial parallels, small circles lying in planes perpendicular to the axis of rotation. This means, of course that the declination of each star remains constant in the course of the diurnal motion, but the hour angle of the star increases (Cf. Fig. 2-4). Both horizontal coordinates of a star

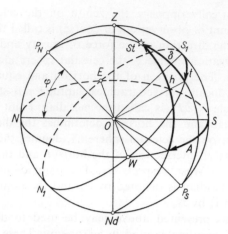

Figure 2-3. The horizon and equatorial-meridian systems of coordinates.

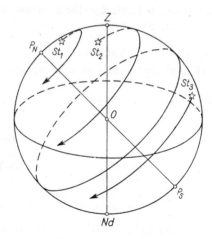

Figure 2-4. The diurnal motion of the celestial sphere.

also change owing to the diurnal motion. Therefore, in specifying the position of some object on the celestial sphere in the horizontal or equatorial-meridian systems we must give the time and place of observation. The latter is done because the position of the horizon and meridian on the celestial sphere depends on the place of observation.

Section 15   The Earth's Orbital Motion Around the Sun

The rotational motion of the Earth discussed in the preceding section provides inducement to introduce a coordinate system such that the position of the object neither varies because of the diurnal motion of the celestial sphere nor depends on the place of observation. In this system both the principal plane P, and the principal direction k would be related to the rotating celestial sphere. Such conditions are met, for instance, in a system in which the equator is the principal plane (the declination of astronomical objects will not change during the diurnal motion of the celestial sphere) and the principal direction is determined by some point on the rotating celestial sphere. The position of some astronomical object cannot be used to determine this point, however since that position on the celestial sphere moves with respect to the Earth. It therefore becomes necessary to determine the principal direction from the dynamic properties of the Earth's motion. If we were to treat the Earth as a sphere and to neglect the influence of other bodies of the solar system, the direction of the Earth's rotational axis and the plane in which the Earth revolves about the Sun would not change. Hence the points common to the celestial equator and the great circle constituting the intersection of the plane of the Earth's motion about the Sun with the celestial sphere, called the ecliptic (the plane of the equator and the ecliptic are at an angle of $\varepsilon = 23°27'$ to each other) would be constant and could be a basis for determining the principal direction in the coordinate system we are seeking. It is true that the assumptions made here are not exact (the Earth is not a sphere, nor can the influence of other bodies of the solar system be neglected), but the factors we have neglected cause only very small motions in the axis and orbital plane of the Earth.

The relative motion of the Earth and the Sun is reflected by the change in the position of the Sun against the background of the stars. The Sun moves amidst the stars on a great circle (whose plane coincides with the plane of relative Earth-Sun motion), executing one complete revolution

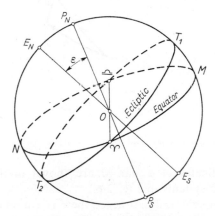

Figure 2-5. The position of the equator and the ecliptic on the celestial sphere. E_N and E_S—the north and south ecliptic poles.

in a time equal to the period of the Earth's revolution around the Sun. The annual motion of the Sun on the ecliptic proceeds from West to East. The points of intersection of the ecliptic with the equator are called equinoctial points. One of them, at which the Sun moves from the Southern to the Northern Hemisphere, is the vernal equinox, also known as the first point of Aries ♈; the one diametrically opposite is the autumnal equinox, the first point of Libra ♎ (Cf. Fig. 2-5).

Table 2-2 presents data characterizing the next two systems of astronomical coordinates: the equatorial-equinoctial system and the ecliptic

TABLE 2-2

Equatorial-equinoctial and Ecliptic Systems

Principal Elements	Equatorial-equinoctial	Ecliptical
Reference plane P	equator	ecliptic
Reference direction **k**	O♈	O♈
Name of angle U	right ascension: α	ecliptic longitude: λ
Direction of increase in angle U	♈**M**♎**N**	♈**T₁**♎**T₂**
Range of angle U	0 to 24ʰ	0 to 360°
Range of angle V	declination: δ	ecliptic latitude: β
Range of angle V	−90 to +90°	−90 to +90°

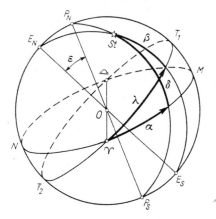

Figure 2-6. Equatorial-equinoctial and ecliptic systems of coordinates.

system. The coordinates of a star St are shown in the equatorial-equinoctial and ecliptic systems in Fig. 2-6.

The Earth is not spherical and hence there is a moment of forces which affects its rotation. The Earth moves in a field of gravitational forces from the Sun, planets, and the Moon. These forces acting on different points of the Earth are not the same; the points of the Earth nearest the attracting body are subjected to the action of a greater force than are points further off. A body of spherical symmetry in such a field moves like a material point with its mass concentrated at the centre of gravity. However, since the equatorial radius of the Earth is greater than its polar

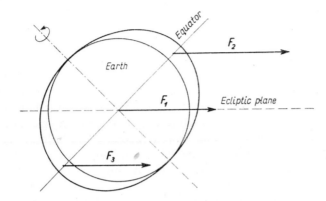

Figure 2-7. The distribution of the Moon's gravitional attraction inside the Earth.

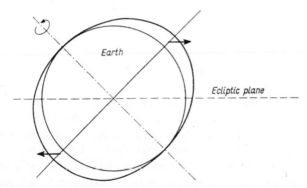

Figure 2-8. The force couple responsible for precession of the Earth's axis.

radius, the existence of a nonuniform gravitational field causes additional dynamic effects. In order to consider these effects qualitatively, we can treat the Earth as an ellipsoid of revolution whose equatorial radius is greater than the polar radius. The forces acting on various parts of the Earth are distributed as shown in Fig. 2-7. (We have assumed here that the interacting body lies on the ecliptic plane.) Part of the forces acting on the Earth is balanced by the centrifugal force resulting from the Earth's motion about the joint centre of gravity of the Earth and the interacting body under consideration. The rest can be described as a couple whose moment is perpendicular to the Earth's axis of rotation (hence, also its angular momentum) at a given instant and lies on the ecliptic plane (Fig. 2-8). Owing to this moment of forces, the axis of the Earth describes a cone of revolution with axis of symmetry perpendicular to the ecliptic plane or, to put it another way, the celestial poles describe on the celestial sphere small circles about the poles of the ecliptic; this phenomenon is called precession. This motion is slow—the celestial pole circles the ecliptic pole once in 26,000 years and, of course, the first point of Aries (vernal equinox) travels around the entire ecliptic in this same time. The first point of Aries precesses East through South to West at $360°/26,000 \approx 50''$ a year. The precession by the Earth's axis is due to the influence primarily of the Moon (because of the proximity of this body to the Earth), secondarily of the Sun and, to a negligible extent, that of the planets.

The inclination of the lunar orbital plane to the ecliptic, as well sa the planetary perturbations in the Earth's motion, cause further motions by the Earth's axis and changes in the position of the equator and the ecliptic on the celestial sphere.

Therefore, whenever the position of a star is given in ecliptic or equatorial-equinoctial systems it is necessary to specify the time of the observation (this time may, however, be given with much less accuracy than when we determine the coordinates of stars in the horizontal or equatorial-meridional systems; why?). Only then can the motion of the ecliptic and the equator be taken into account in order to calculate the coordinates of that star at any instant.

Hitherto we have considered the relative motion of the Earth and the Sun, as evidenced by the annual motion of the Sun on the ecliptic. From the point of view of dynamics (neglecting the effect of other bodies of the solar system) the motion of the Sun and the Earth should be regarded as motion about a common centre of mass. Since the Sun is vastly more massive than the Earth, this centre lies much closer to the centre of the Sun (in fact, it lies deep inside the Sun) than to the centre of the Earth. The radius of the Earth's orbit is consequently much greater than that of the Sun's orbit and this motion may, in the first approximation, be treated as the Earth circling a stationary Sun. This conclusion can be drawn from dynamical considerations. However, observational proof of the Earth's orbiting motion does exist. This proof is provided by what is called the parallactic shift of the stars. Because the Earth orbits the Sun, the direction at which a star is seen from various points on the Earth's orbit changes with time (Cf. Fig. 2-9). The star describes on the celestial sphere an ellipse whose major semiaxis (parallel to the ecliptic), called the stellar parallax, is expressed in seconds by

$$\pi = 206{,}265''a/r, \qquad (2\text{-}1)$$

a) b)

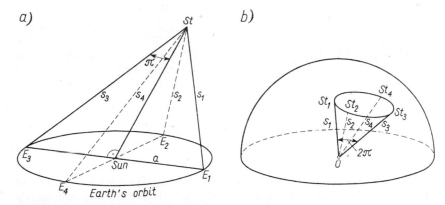

Figure 2-9. Parallax: a) the directions s_1, s_2, s_3, s_4 at which we see star St from four points E_1, E_2, E_3, E_4 of the Earth's orbit around the Sun; b) the positions St_1, St_2, St_3, St_4 (and the parallactic ellipse drawn through them) from the Earth E of the star St on the celestial sphere at the same instants as in (a). Of course, the observer O is at the centre of the celestial sphere.

where a is the semi-major axis of the Earth's orbit, and r is the distance to the star, given in the same units as a. The method of determining the distance of stars from Eq. (2-1) is called the method of trigonometrical parallaxes.

Because the parallax depends on the distance of the star from the Earth (Sun), the parallaxes of distant stars are so small that the errors of measurement become greater than the parallaxes themselves. Measurements of trigonometric parallaxes can thus be used to determine the distances of only the closest stars (even then the parallaxes amount to mere fractions of a second of arc), whereas distances to more distant stars must be found by other methods.

Equation (2-1) can be used to associate two different units of length employed in astronomy. One of them is the astronomical unit, AU, which is equal to the semi-major axis of the Earth's orbit. The length of the astronomical unit (Cf. Sec. 20) is 1.496×10^{13} cm, or 149,600,000 km (92,960,000 mi). The distances of bodies in the solar system are in general expressed in terms of astronomical units. The other unit of length which we use to express the distance of stars is the parsec. The parsec (pc) is equal to the distance of an object whose parallax is $1''$. By Eq. (2-1) we have

$$1 \text{ pc} = 206,265 \text{ AU} = 3.0857 \times 10^{18} \text{ cm} = 3.0857 \times 10^{13} \text{ km}.$$

Also used are derivative units of the parsec, that is, the kiloparsec and the megaparsec.

1 kiloparsec = 1 kpc = 10^3 pc = 3.0857×10^{21} cm = 3.0857×10^{16} km,

1 megaparsec = 1 Mpc = 10^6 pc = 3.0857×10^{24} cm = 3.0857×10^{19} km.

Independent proof of the Earth's orbital motion is provided by observations of the aberration of star light. If observers who are moving with respect to each other at non-zero velocity make observations from the same place, they see the same source of light in somewhat different apparent directions. An observer on the Earth moves with a velocity which changes direction and, consequently, the apparent direction of the light source changes; in a year the star describes an aberration ellipse in the sky.

The positions of stars on the celestial sphere also vary as a result of the motion of the stars with respect to the Sun. If a star has a nonvanishing component of velocity with respect to the Sun, perpendicular to the Sun-star direction, the star is displaced on the celestial sphere. This displacement, expressed in units of angle per year, is called the proper motion μ. If the distance r of the star is known from other sources, its proper motion enables us to find the tangential component V_t of its velocity which is perpendicular to the direction Sun-star:

$$V_t = kr\mu, \tag{2-2}$$

where k is a constant introduced in order to convert the units adopted (if μ is expressed in seconds of arc per year, V_t in kilometres per second, and r in parsec, then $k \approx 4.74$).

Section 16   Astronomical Time

The motion of the celestial sphere is utilized to define astronomical units of time. The fundamental unit here is the sidereal day, the interval between two successive meridian passages of the vernal equinox. The sidereal day is divided into 24 sidereal hours. In turn, each sidereal hour consists of 60 sidereal minutes, and each of these has 60 sidereal seconds. In a given locality, the sidereal day begins when the vernal equinox is on the local meridian.

Thus, as follows from the above, sidereal time ϑ is measured by the motion of the vernal equinox. Namely

$$\vartheta = t_\varphi, \tag{2-3}$$

where t_φ is the hour angle of the vernal equinox. Since, for any star, we have

$$t_\varphi = t + \alpha \tag{2-4}$$

(where α is the right ascension and t the hour angle of the star), therefore

$$\vartheta = t + \alpha \tag{2-5}$$

that is, the sidereal time in a given locality is the sum of the hour angle and the right ascension of any astronomical object. It follows from Eq. (2-5) that the sidereal time is equal to the right ascension of an ascending star (in transit through the meridian at that instant), since $t = 0$ for that star.

It would be inconvenient to use sidereal time in everyday life since the sidereal day begins at various times throughout the day owing to the annual motion of the Sun on the ecliptic. Consequently, mean solar time is used in addition to sidereal time. In determining the mean solar time, we employ an auxiliary concept of the mean Sun. This is taken to be a mathematical point executing annual motion along the celestial equator with constant angular velocity in the same direction the Sun moves on the ecliptic. The introduction of the mean Sun in place of the actual position of the Sun is necessary for two reasons. First, the Sun traces its annual orbit on the ecliptic, and not the celestial equator. Second, the motion of the Sun on the ecliptic is not uniform, inasmuch as the Earth moves in an elliptical orbit with variable velocity. For both of these reasons, the right ascension of the true Sun does not move uniformly.

The unit of mean solar time is the mean solar day. This is the interval of time which elapses between two successive meridian passages of the mean Sun. The mean solar day is divided into mean solar hours, minutes, and seconds. The mean solar day begins when the mean Sun makes its downward meridian passage, that is, when the hour angle of the mean Sun is 12^h. Hence the mean solar time

$$t_m = t_{\odot m} - 12^h, \qquad (2\text{-}6)$$

where $t_{\odot m}$ is the hour angle of the mean Sun.

Since the mean solar time is measured by the hour angle of the mean Sun, at any given instant this time is different at any two points on the Earth with different geographical longitudes. This has led to the introduction of zone time which, within a given zone, differs by an integral number of hours from the universal time, i.e. from the mean solar time on the Greenwich meridian ($0°$ geographical longitude). The boundaries between zones run roughly along meridians which correspond to geographical longitudes of $7° 30' \pm n \cdot 15°$ (where n is a natural number), in general taking account of the shape of international boundaries. Central European Time which is in effect in Poland, for instance, is one hour ahead of universal time.

The annual motion of the Sun on the ecliptic is the base on which a larger unit of time is defined. This is the tropical year, defined as the interval between two successive transits of the Sun through the vernal equinox. The tropical year is equal to $365^d 5^h 48^m 46^s$, or 365.2422 mean solar days. Since the calendar used for practical purposes must have a whole number of days in the year, calendar years of various lengths had to be introduced: ordinary years of 365 mean solar days and leap years of 366 days. The Gregorian calendar, which was introduced in the 16th century, is now used nearly everywhere. In this calendar, every year divisible by four is a leap year, except for century years which must be divisible by 400 in order to be a leap year. According to the Gregorian calendar, the average year is 365.2425 mean solar days in length and is only about 26^s longer than the tropical year.

Note, however, that the tropical year, which is the period when the cyclical seasons of the year recur (why?) and was for this reason used as a basis for establishing the length of the calendar year, is not equal to the period of the Earth's revolution about the Sun. Indeed, the length of the tropical year is determined by using the concept of the vernal equinox which, as we know from the preceding section, moves on the ecliptic. In consequence, the period of the Earth's revolution about the Sun, called the sidereal year, is somewhat longer than the tropical year, namely, is $365^d\ 6^h\ 9^m\ 10^s$, or 365.2564 mean solar days.

Chapter 3   The Physics of the Solar System

THE MECHANICS OF THE SOLAR SYSTEM

The motion of bodies in the solar system is governed by the field of the gravitational forces of the Sun and the planets. The mutual gravitational attractions of the planetoids, comets, and interplanetary matter may be neglected since their mass is negligible compared to the mass of the entire system. All of the planets and their moons, as well as the Sun, are nearly spherical bodies. The deviations of their surfaces from the spherical are so small in comparison with the distances between the planets that in most problems in the mechanics of the solar system the gravitational field may be treated as originating from a system of particles or material points.

In considering the motion of the massive members of the solar system—the planets, their moons, and the planetoids—we may neglect the influence of nongravitational forces—such as radiation pressure, the magnetic field of the Sun and the planets, and the aerodynamic resistance of the interplanetary medium—which have a major effect on the dynamics of diffused interplanetary matter. For these reasons, in the sections below we shall confine ourselves to a study of the behaviour of a system of n particles (material points) linked together by mutual gravitational attractions.

Section 17   The n-body Problem

Let us consider a system of n particles of masses m_i $(i = 1, 2, ..., n)$. By $[x_i, y_i, z_i] = \mathbf{r}_i$ we denote the radius vector of the i-th point in any inertial system of rectilinear coordinates XYZ. Let us assume that each pair of particles attract each other with a force given by Newton's law

$$\mathbf{F}_{ij} = -G \frac{m_i m_j}{r_{ij}^3} \mathbf{r}_{ij}, \quad \text{when} \quad i \neq j$$

and

$$\mathbf{F}_{ii} = 0, \tag{3-1}$$

where $\mathbf{r}_{ij} = \mathbf{r}_i - \mathbf{r}_j = [x_i - x_j, y_i - y_j, z_i - z_j]$, $\mathbf{F}_{ij}$ is the force with which particle j attracts particle i, and $G = 6.670 \times 10^{-8}$ cm$^3 \cdot$ g$^{-1} \cdot$ sec^{-2} is the gravitational constant.

The motion of particle i is described by the equation

$$m_i \ddot{\mathbf{r}}_i = \sum_{j=1}^{n} \mathbf{F}_{ij}, \quad i = 1, 2, ..., n, \tag{3-2}$$

where a dot over a symbol indicates a derivative with respect to time.

Let us take the sum of Eq. (3-2) over i

$$\sum_{i=1}^{n} m_i \ddot{\mathbf{r}}_i = \sum_{i=1}^{n} \sum_{j=1}^{n} \mathbf{F}_{ij}. \tag{3-3}$$

Since by Eq. (3-1) we have

$$\mathbf{F}_{ij} = -\mathbf{F}_{ji}, \tag{3-4}$$

whence

$$\sum_{i=1}^{n} \sum_{j=1}^{n} \mathbf{F}_{ij} = 0 \tag{3-5}$$

and Eq. (3-3) simplifies to

$$\sum_{i=1}^{n} m_i \ddot{\mathbf{r}}_i = 0. \tag{3-6}$$

Integrating Eq. (3-6) twice over time, we obtain

$$\sum_{i=1}^{n} m_i \mathbf{r}_i = \mathbf{a}t + \mathbf{b}, \tag{3-7}$$

where $\mathbf{a}$ and $\mathbf{b}$ are arbitrary constant vectors.

It follows from Eq. (3-7) that the centre of mass of a system whose radius vector is specified by

$$\mathbf{r}_0 = \frac{\displaystyle\sum_{i=1}^{n} m_i \mathbf{r}_i}{\displaystyle\sum_{i=1}^{n} m_i} \tag{3-8}$$

moves with constant velocity along a straight line. The potential energy of the system is a function of the coordinates of the particles—and through them, a function of time; it is given by

$$U = U\big(x_1(t), y_1(t), z_1(t), \dots, x_n(t), y_n(t), z_n(t)\big)$$

$$= -\tfrac{1}{2} G \sum_{k=1}^{n} \sum_{\substack{l=1 \\ l \neq k}}^{n} \frac{m_k m_l}{r_{kl}}. \tag{3-9}$$

Differentiating Eq. (3-9) partially with respect to x_i, y_i, z_i, we can show that

$$-\sum_{j=1}^{n} \mathbf{F}_{ij} = \left[\frac{\partial U}{\partial x_i}, \frac{\partial U}{\partial y_i}, \frac{\partial U}{\partial z_i} \right]. \tag{3-10}$$

Thus, Eq. (3) can be rewritten as

$$m_i \ddot{x}_i = -\frac{\partial U}{\partial x_i},$$

$$m_i \ddot{y}_i = -\frac{\partial U}{\partial y_i}, \qquad (3\text{-}11)$$

$$m_i \ddot{z}_i = -\frac{\partial U}{\partial z_i}.$$

When we multiply the first equation of Eq. (3-11) by $\dot{x}_i$, the second by $\dot{y}_i$, and the third by $\dot{z}_i$, add by sides, and take the sum over i, the result is

$$\sum_{i=1}^{n} m_i(\ddot{x}_i \dot{x}_i + \ddot{y}_i \dot{y}_i + \ddot{z}_i \dot{z}_i) = -\sum_{i=1}^{n} \left(\frac{\partial U}{\partial x_i} \dot{x}_i + \frac{\partial U}{\partial y_i} \dot{y}_i + \frac{\partial U}{\partial z_i} \dot{z}_i \right) = -\frac{dU}{dt}.$$

$$(3\text{-}12)$$

Since

$$(\ddot{x}_i \dot{x}_i + \ddot{y}_i \dot{y}_i + \ddot{z}_i \dot{z}_i) = \tfrac{1}{2} \frac{d}{dt} [\dot{x}_i^2 + \dot{y}_i^2 + \dot{z}_i^2] \qquad (3\text{-}13)$$

integration of Eq. (3-12) yields

$$\tfrac{1}{2} \sum_{i=1}^{n} m_i(\dot{x}_i^2 + \dot{y}_i^2 + \dot{z}_i^2) + U = h, \qquad (3\text{-}14)$$

where h is a constant of integration.

Equation (3-14), called the energy integral, expresses the law: the sum of the kinetic and potential energy of an isolated system remains constant.

Now, let us multiply both sides of Eq. (3-2) vectorially by $\mathbf{r}_i$ and take the sum over all particles,

$$\sum_{i=1}^{n} m_i \mathbf{r}_i \times \ddot{\mathbf{r}}_i = \sum_{i=1}^{n} \mathbf{r}_i \times \sum_{j=1}^{n} \mathbf{F}_{ij} = -\sum_{i=1}^{n} \sum_{\substack{j=1 \\ j \neq i}}^{n} \mathbf{r}_i \times G \frac{m_i m_j}{r_{ij}^3} \mathbf{r}_{ij}$$

$$= -\sum_{i=1}^{n} \sum_{\substack{j=1 \\ j \neq i}}^{n} G \frac{m_i m_j}{r_{ij}^3} [\mathbf{r}_i \times (\mathbf{r}_i - \mathbf{r}_j)] = \sum_{i=1}^{n} \sum_{\substack{j=1 \\ j \neq i}}^{n} G \frac{m_i m_j}{r_{ij}^3} \mathbf{r}_i \times \mathbf{r}_j. \qquad (3\text{-}15)$$

To each pair of particles (labelled k and l, for instance) there correspond in the expression $\displaystyle\sum_{i=1}^{n} \sum_{\substack{j=1 \\ j \neq i}}^{n} G \frac{m_i m_j}{r_{ij}^3} \mathbf{r}_i \times \mathbf{r}_j$ two vectors $G \dfrac{m_k m_l}{r_{kl}^3} \mathbf{r}_l \times \mathbf{r}_k$ and $G \dfrac{m_k m_l}{r_{lk}^3} \mathbf{r}_k \times \mathbf{r}_l$, which differ only in sense. Therefore their sum is zero and the right-hand side of Eq. (15) thus vanishes. Hence

$$\sum_{i=1}^{n} m_i \mathbf{r}_i \times \ddot{\mathbf{r}}_i = 0. \tag{3-16}$$

Since

$$\mathbf{r}_i \times \ddot{\mathbf{r}}_i = \frac{d}{dt} (\mathbf{r}_i \times \dot{\mathbf{r}}_i) \tag{3-17}$$

consequently

$$\frac{d}{dt} \left(\sum_{i=1}^{n} m_i \mathbf{r}_i \times \dot{\mathbf{r}}_i \right) = 0. \tag{3-18}$$

Upon integration of Eq. (18), we obtain

$$\sum_{i=1}^{n} m_i \mathbf{r}_i \times \dot{\mathbf{r}}_i = \mathbf{c}. \tag{3-19}$$

This equation means that the total angular momentum of the system is constant.

When we rewite Eq. (3-19) in terms of the coordinates, we have

$$\sum_{i=1}^{n} m_i (y_i \dot{z}_i - z_i \dot{y}_i) = c_1, \tag{3-20}$$

$$\sum_{i=1}^{n} m_i (z_i \dot{x}_i - x_i \dot{z}_i) = c_2, \tag{3-21}$$

$$\sum_{i=1}^{n} m_i (x_i \dot{y}_i - y_i \dot{x}_i) = c_3. \tag{3-22}$$

Equations (3-20)–(3-22) are known as areal integrals. Vector $\mathbf{c}$, whose respective coordinates constitute the right-hand sides of Eqs. (3-20)–(3-22) is constant. The plane normal to that vector and passing through the centre of mass is called the invariable plane of the system.

Thus we have ten first integrals describing the motion of a system of n particles: 6 integrals describing the motion of the centre of mass (3 components of vector $\mathbf{a}$ and 3 of vector $\mathbf{b}$)—Eq. (3-7), an energy integral—Eq. (3-14), and 3 integrals of area—Eqs. (3-20)–(3-22). Since the motion of each particle is determined by a set of 3 scalar differential equations of the second order (3-2), we must know $6n$ integrals of motion in order to obtain a general solution for the n-body problem.

Unfortunately, in the general case single-valued integrals of motion apart from those given above do not exist. For this reason, the n-body problem is insoluble analytically.

Using the energy integral, we can formulate the following theorem: If the total energy of a system of n particles is negative ($h < 0$), there exist at least two bodies of that system which cannot move apart from each other to an infinite distance.

Proof

Since the kinetic energy of the system cannot be negative by Eqs. (3-14) and (3-9) we can write

$$\frac{1}{2} G \sum_{i=1}^{n} \sum_{\substack{j=1 \\ j \neq i}}^{n} \frac{m_i m_j}{r_{ij}} > -h > 0. \tag{3-23}$$

If the distance between each pair of bodies tended to infinity, the expression

$$\frac{1}{2} G \sum_{i=1}^{n} \sum_{\substack{j=1 \\ j \neq i}}^{n} \frac{m_i m_j}{r_{ij}}$$

would tend to zero and, from a certain instant, would become smaller than some arbitrary, positive number $\varepsilon < -h$, but this is in contradiction with inequality (3-23).

Conclusion: If the total energy of an isolated system of two bodies is negative, the system is stable, i.e. there exists a distance d such that always

$$r_{12} < d. \tag{3-24}$$

Section 18 The Two-body Problem

The motion of two bodies is completely specified when $6 \times 2 = 12$ integrals are given. Ten first integrals were obtained in the preceding section. In the present section we shall find the two missing integrals of motion for two particles. We shall thus obtain a general, analytical solution of the two-body problem.

The equations of motion for a system of n particles were written in some arbitrary inertial frame. The centre of mass of the system moves uniformly in space in a straight line, Eq. (3-7). The reference frame can thus be moved so that its origin is at the centre of mass. The reference frame so introduced is also inertial and, therefore, all of our integrals are of the same form in this frame.

Equations (3-7) simplifies to

$$m_1 \mathbf{r}_1 + m_2 \mathbf{r}_2 = 0, \tag{3-25}$$

whence $\mathbf{r}_1 \| \mathbf{r}_2$, and Eq. (3-19) can be rewritten as

$$\mathbf{c} = m_1 \mathbf{r}_1 \times \dot{\mathbf{r}}_1 + m_2 \mathbf{r}_2 \times \dot{\mathbf{r}}_2. \tag{3-26}$$

Multiplication of both sides of Eq. (3-26) scal rly by $\mathbf{r}_i$ $(i = 1, 2)$ yields

$$\mathbf{c} \cdot \mathbf{r}_i = m_1 (\mathbf{r}_1 \times \dot{\mathbf{r}}_1) \cdot \mathbf{r}_i + m_2 (\mathbf{r}_2 \times \dot{\mathbf{r}}_2) \cdot \mathbf{r}_i \tag{3-27}$$

and since $(\mathbf{r}_1 \times \dot{\mathbf{r}}_1) \perp \mathbf{r}_i$ and $(\mathbf{r}_2 \times \dot{\mathbf{r}}_2) \perp \mathbf{r}_i$, therefore

$$\mathbf{c} \cdot \mathbf{r}_i = 0. \tag{3-28}$$

By virtue of Eq. (3-28) we can formulate the theorem:

The motion of two bodies takes place in a fixed plane passing through the centre of mass (in the invariable plane of the system).

Since, by Eq. (3-25)

$$\mathbf{r}_1 = - \frac{m_2}{m_1 + m_2} \mathbf{r} \tag{3-29}$$

and

$$\mathbf{r}_2 = \frac{m_1}{m_1 + m_2} \mathbf{r}, \tag{3-30}$$

where

$$\mathbf{r} = \mathbf{r}_2 - \mathbf{r}_1 = \mathbf{r}_{21} \tag{3-31}$$

is a vector running from the body of mass m_1 to mass m_2, the energy integral (3-14) can be rewritten as

$$\dot{\mathbf{r}}^2 - 2G \frac{m_1 + m_2}{r} = h', \tag{3-32}$$

where h' is a new constant $\left(h' = 2 \frac{m_1 + m_2}{m_1 m_2} h \right)$. Similarly the areal integral can be brought to the form

$$\mathbf{r} \times \dot{\mathbf{r}} = \mathbf{c}', \tag{3-33}$$

where $\mathbf{c}'$ is a constant vector $\left(\mathbf{c}' = \frac{m_1 + m_2}{m_1 m_2} \mathbf{c} \right)$.

Half the length of the vector $\mathbf{r} \times \dot{\mathbf{r}}$ is called the areal velocity and is equal to the area swept per unit time by the vector drawn from the particle of mass m_1 to the particle of mass m_2. By Eq. (3-33) we can state the theorem:

The relative motion of two bodies proceeds with constant areal velocity.

This statement constitutes the essence of Kepler's third law.

Let us now introduce a system of polar coordinates (r, θ, z) with origin at the particle of mass m_1, and the Z-axis oriented in some arbitrary direction in the invariable plane of the system. Simple manipulation gives

$$\dot{\mathbf{r}}^2 = \dot{r}^2 + r^2 \dot{\theta}^2 \tag{3-34}$$

and

$$|\mathbf{r} \times \mathbf{r}| = r^2 \dot{\theta}. \tag{3-35}$$

The set of Eqs. (3-32) and (3-33) yields a new integral of motion for two bodies. Substitution of Eqs. (3-34) and (3-35) in them gives

$$\dot{r}^2 + r^2 \dot{\theta}^2 - 2 \frac{\mu}{r} = h' \tag{3-36}$$

and

$$r^2 \dot{\theta} = c', \tag{3-37}$$

where

$$\mu = G(m_1 + m_2). \tag{3-38}$$

Since

$$\dot{r} = \frac{dr}{d\theta}\dot{\theta} = \frac{dr}{d\theta}r^{-2}c' \tag{3-39}$$

then Eq. (3-37) can be used to rewrite Eq. (3-36) in the form

$$\left[\frac{dr}{d\theta}r^{-2}\right]^2 + r^{-2} - 2\frac{\mu}{c'^2}r^{-1} = \frac{h'}{c'^2}. \tag{3-40}$$

We introduce the notations

$$p = \frac{c'^2}{\mu}, \tag{3-41}$$

$$e = \left[1 + \frac{c'^2 h'}{\mu^2}\right]^{\frac{1}{2}}, \tag{3-42}$$

$$\frac{1}{r} = \frac{1}{p}(1 + eu), \tag{3-43}$$

where u is a new variable. Substituting Eqs. (3-41)–(3-43) in Eq. (3-40), we obtain

$$\left[\frac{du}{d\theta}\right]^2 + u^2 - 1 = 0 \tag{3-44}$$

whence

$$-\frac{du}{\sqrt{1-u^2}} = d\theta. \tag{3-45}$$

When we integrate the above equations, we arrive at

$$\arccos u = \theta - \theta_0, \tag{3-46}$$

where $\theta_0 = $ const. In this manner we have obtained the next, eleventh integral of motion for two bodies. Equation (3-46) yields

$$u = \cos(\theta - \theta_0) \tag{3-47}$$

whence

$$r = \frac{p}{1 + e\cos(\theta - \theta_0)}. \tag{3-48}$$

Equation (3-48)* describes in polar coordinates curves which are conic

* The second root of Eq. (3-44)

$$\frac{du}{\sqrt{1-u^2}} = d\theta \tag{3-45'}$$

leads to the solution

$$r = \frac{p}{1 + e\sin(\theta - \theta_1)} \tag{3-48'}$$

where θ_1 is a constant of integration. Equations (3-48) and (3-48') describe the same curve when the substitution $\theta_1 = \theta_0 - 90°$ is made.

sections—ellipse $(e < 1)$, parabola $(e = 1)$, hyperbola $(e > 1)$—with one focus at the origin of the system. On the basis of this equation, we can formulate what is known as Kepler's first law:

When two bodies, linked only by gravitational forces, are in relative motion with respect to each other, each of them moves along a conic section which has the other body at its focus.

The motion of a body of mass m_2 relative to a body mass m_1 will be completely determined if we find a relation which gives the position of the body in its orbit as a function of time. In order to find this relation, the

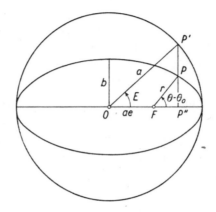

Figure 3-1. The elements of the ellipse: *a*—semimajor axis, *b*—semi-minor axis, *O*—centre of ellipse, *F*—focus at which the central body is located, $\theta - \theta_0$—the true anomaly, *E*—the eccentric anomaly.

cases of elliptic, parabolic, and hyperbolic orbits should be considered separately. Only the case of elliptic orbits will be discussed in any detail here.

From analytical geometry we know the relations (Cf. Fig. 3-1)

$$\frac{PP''}{P'P''} = \frac{b}{a} = (1-e^2)^{1/2}, \tag{3-49}$$

$$a = p(1-e^2)^{-1}. \tag{3-50}$$

Since

$$PP'' = r\sin(\theta-\theta_0), \quad P'P'' = a\sin E, \\ FP'' = r\cos(\theta-\theta_0), \quad OP'' = a\cos E \tag{3-51}$$

therefore

$$r\sin(\theta-\theta_0) = a(1-e^2)^{1/2}\sin E, \tag{3-52}$$

$$r\cos(\theta-\theta_0) = a(\cos E-e). \tag{3-53}$$

Dividing Eqs. (52) and (53) by sides, we obtain

$$\tan(\theta-\theta_0) = \frac{\sin E}{\cos E-e} (1-e^2)^{1/2} \qquad (3\text{-}54)$$

whence, by differentiation, we have

$$\cos^{-2}(\theta-\theta_0)\,d\theta = -\frac{1-e\cos E}{(\cos E-e)^2} (1-e^2)^{1/2}dE. \qquad (3\text{-}55)$$

Using the areal integrals (3-37) and Eq. (3-55), we can write

$$c'dt = r^2d\theta = r^2\cos^2(\theta-\theta_0)\frac{1-e\cos E}{(\cos E-e)^2} (1-e^2)^{1/2}dE. \qquad (3\text{-}56)$$

When Eq. (3-53) is taken into consideration we obtain

$$\frac{c'}{a^2(1-e^2)^{1/2}} \, dt = (1-e\cos E)\,dE \qquad (3\text{-}57)$$

whence

$$n(t-t_0) = E-e\sin E, \qquad (3\text{-}58)$$

where

$$n = \frac{c'}{a^2(1-e^2)^{1/2}} = \frac{\mu^{1/2}p^{1/2}(1-e^2)^{-1/2}}{a^2} = \frac{\mu^{1/2}a^{1/2}}{a^2} = \frac{\sqrt{G(m_1+m_2)}}{a^{3/2}} \qquad (3\text{-}59)$$

is called the mean diurnal motion, and t_0 is a constant of integration*. Equation (3-58) is called Kepler's equation and is the twelfth and last integral of motion of two bodies. The eccentric anomaly E can be found from Kepler's equation for any given time t and Eqs. (3-52) and (3-53) can then be used to find the true anomaly $\theta-\theta_0$.

By $\mathscr{P}$ let us denote the period in which the body of mass m_1 circles the

---

* The corresponding equation for motion in a parabolic orbit is of the form

$$\tan\tfrac{1}{2}(\theta-\theta_0)+\tfrac{1}{3}\tan^3\tfrac{1}{2}(\theta-\theta_0)=2\frac{\mu^2}{c'^3}(t-t_0)$$

and for motion in a hyperbola

$$e\tan F-\ln\tan(45°+\tfrac{1}{2}F)=n(t-t_0),$$

where

$$\tan\tfrac{1}{2}(\theta-\theta_0) = \left(\frac{e+1}{e-1}\right)^{1/2}\tan\tfrac{1}{2}F.$$

body of mass m_2. During the period $\mathscr{P}$ the left-hand side of Eq. (3-58) increases by nP, and the right-hand side, by 2π. Thus

$$n\mathscr{P} = 2\pi. \tag{3-60}$$

Using the definition of n, we have

$$\sqrt{G(m_1+m_2)}\;\frac{\mathscr{P}}{a^{3/2}} = 2\pi \tag{3-61}$$

whence

$$\frac{a^3}{\mathscr{P}^2} = \frac{G(m_1+m_2)}{4\pi^2}. \tag{3-62}$$

The equation above constitutes the essence of Kepler's third law:

The ratio of the cube of the semimajor axis of the orbit to the square of the period of revolution is proportional to the sum of the masses of both bodies.

Kepler's laws originally had a different, somewhat more restricted formulation. At a time when Newton had not yet presented the law of universal gravitation, Kepler formulated these laws as follows on the basis of his observations of planetary motions:

First Law (The Law of Orbits): Each planet moves about the Sun in an orbit that is an ellipse, with the Sun at one focus of the ellipse.

Second Law (The Law of Areas): The straight line joining a planet and the Sun sweeps out equal areas in space in equal intervals of time.

Third Law (Harmonic Law): The squares of the sidereal periods of the planets are in direct proportion to the cubes of the semimajor axes of their orbits.

Section 19   The Orbits of Planets and Comets

The planets move about the Sun in the common gravitational field of the Sun and the planets. However, the masses of the planets are small in comparison to the solar mass and their orbits are such that the distances between the planets are considerable. Hence, in the first approximation the interaction of the planets with each other can be neglected and their motion may be assumed to take place only in the gravitational field of the Sun. In this case, at any instant the position of any planet with respect to a chosen plane E moving in space together with the Sun is specified by means of the six integrals of motion obtained for two bodies in the preceding section—h', c_1', c_2', c_3', θ_0, t_0, where c_1', c_2', c_3', are the components of the vector $\mathbf{c}'$, in a reference frame fixed in the plane E.

Usually, however, the positions of planets are specified by means of other parameters—called orbital elements (Fig. 3-2, Table 3-1)—which have a simple geometric sense. The plane of the ecliptic, in which the direction to the vernal equinox point is treated as the principal direction, is taken as plane E; the angle θ is measured in the orbital plane from the direction to the ascending node.

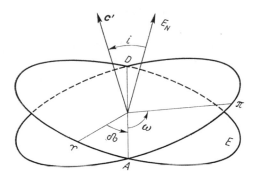

Figure 3-2. The elements of an orbit: E—ecliptic plane, ♈—vernal equi-nox point, A—ascending node, D—descending node, π—perihelion (the point on the orbit closest to the Sun), i—inclination of orbit, ☊—longitude of ascending node, ω—distance of perihelion from node.

TABLE 3-1

The Elements of an Orbit

Symbol	Name	Expressed by Integrals of Motion
a	Semimajor axis	$a = -\dfrac{\mu}{h'}$
e	Eccentricity	$e = \left[1 + \dfrac{|\mathbf{c}'|^2 h'}{\mu^2}\right]^{\frac{1}{2}}$
i	Inclination of the orbital plane	$\cos i = c_3' |\mathbf{c}'|^{-1}$
☊	Longitude of the ascending node	$\tan ☊ = -\dfrac{c_1'}{c_2'}$
ω	Argument of perihelion	$\omega = \theta_0$
T_0	Time of perihelion passage	$T_0 = t_0$

In the case of parabolic orbits $a = \infty$. Therefore, the distance of the periphelion from the Sun, $q = |\mathbf{c}'|^2 / 2\mu$, is used instead of the semimajor axis for parabolic orbits.

Inasmuch as they are functions only of the first integrals, the orbital elements a, e, i, ☊, ω, T_0 are time-invariant if the perturbing influence of the planets in the motion is disregarded. In actual fact, the orbital elements undergo slow variations which we can calculate at any moment, provided we know the configuration of the planets. These variations are slight for the planetary orbits. On the other hand, the perturbations in the motion of comets and planetoids, especially those which approach Jupiter (or some other planet) in their revolution about the Sun, may lead to pronounced changes in the orbital elements.

In order to calculate the six orbital elements we must determine by observation at least six numbers specifying the position and motion of bodies on the celestial sphere. We can do this by observing the right ascension α and declination δ of a given body at three different instants. In practice, we make many more observations. The orbital elements so determined have smaller observational errors than they would if found only from three observations of α and δ.

TABLE 3-2

The Elements of the Planetary Orbits (Jan. 1, 1972)

Planet	a (AU)	e	i	☊	ω
Mercury	0.38710	0.20563	7° 0′ 15″	47° 59′ 58″	29° 1′ 12″
Venus	0.72333	0.00679	3° 23′ 40″	76° 25′ 40″	54° 44′ 58″
Earth	1.00000	0.01672	0°	—	101° 13′ 15″
Mars	1.52369	0.09338	1° 50′ 59″	49° 20′ 30″	286° 12′ 7″
Jupiter	5.2032	0.04812	1° 18′ 21″	100° 9′ 51″	273° 37′ 25″
Saturn	9.5162	0.05290	2° 29′ 21″	113° 26′ 3″	339° 39′ 41″
Uranus	19.2379	0.04889	0° 46′ 23″	73° 51′ 59″	99° 4′ 46″
Neptune	30.2159	0.00471	1° 46′ 20″	131° 29′ 5″	247° 45′ 12″
Pluto	39.6007	0.25217	17° 8′ 53″	110° 2′ 11″	113° 34′ 59″

Section 20   The Distances, Masses, and Diameters of the Planets

In determining the orbit of a planet only from observations of the planet on the celestial sphere (that is, by using only angular data), we cannot obtain the semimajor axis of the orbit in absolute units, but rather the ratio of the semimajor axis to that of the Earth's orbit. In other words, we can calculate the length of the semimajor axis in astronomical units. It is a separate matter to find the length of the astronomical unit and use it to express the semimajor axis of the orbit in kilometres. Similarly, from measurements of the positions of a planet's moons during their motion about the planet we can calculate the radii of their orbits (in astronomical units). Knowledge of these relative distances, however, is sufficient for determining the ratios of the planetary masses to the solar mass.

Denote the masses of the Sun, a planet, and one of the latter's satellites by M, m_1, and m_2, respectively; the semimajor axis of the satellite's orbit and its period of revolution about the planet by a_1 and $\mathscr{P}_1$; and the semimajor axis of the planet's orbit and its period of revolution about the Sun by a_2 and $\mathscr{P}_2$. Then, by Kepler's Third Law (3-62), we can write

$$\frac{a_1^3}{\mathscr{P}_1^2} = \frac{G(M+m_1)}{4\pi^2} \tag{3-63}$$

and

$$\frac{a_2^3}{\mathscr{P}_2^2} = \frac{G(m_1+m_2)}{4\pi^2}.$$ (3-64)

Dividing Eqs. (3-63) and (3-64) by sides, we have

$$\left(\frac{a_2}{a_1}\right)^3 \left(\frac{\mathscr{P}_1}{\mathscr{P}_2}\right)^2 = \frac{m_1+m_2}{M+m_1}.$$ (3-65)

When we neglect the planetary mass m_1 as small in comparison to the solar mass M, and the satellite mass m_2 in comparison to the planetary m_1, we arrive at

$$\frac{m_1}{M} = \left(\frac{a_2}{a_1}\right)^3 \left(\frac{\mathscr{P}_1}{\mathscr{P}_2}\right)^2.$$ (3-66)

Equation (3-66) contains only the ratio of the semimajor axes a_1 and a_2 which, therefore, need not be known in absolute units. Since the periods of revolution are also known from observation, the ratio of the planetary to solar mass can be found from Eq. (3-66). Inasmuch as gravimetric measurements give us the mass of the Earth (5.975×10^{27} g), we can use Eq. (3-66) to calculate the solar mass (1.991×10^{33} g) and then the planetary masses. The masses of planets which have no moons are found from the perturbation which these planets cause in the motion of other bodies of the solar system.

Determination of the astronomical unit is based on knowledge of the distance (in kilometres) between any two bodies of the solar system. It was for this purpose that the positions of a given body (most frequently the nearest planets—Venus and Mars, or one of the planetoids) on the celestial sphere were measured from two points on Earth. The angle between the directions to the given celestial body is directly proportional to the known

TABLE 3-3

Masses, Diameters, and Mean Densities of the Planets

Planets	No. of Moons	Mass (Earth = 1)	Diameter (Earth = 1)	Mean Density (g/cm³)
Mercury	—	5.3×10^{-2}	0.40	4.6
Venus	—	8.2×10^{-1}	0.99	4.6
Earth	1	1	1	5.5
Mars	2	0.11	0.54	3.9
Jupiter	12	318	11	1.3
Saturn	10	95	9	0.7
Uranus	5	15	4.2	1.1
Neptune	2	17	3.9	1.6
Pluto	—	0.9?	?	?

distance between the observation points and inversely proportional to the distance of the given body. This made it possible to find the distance of the given body from the Earth in kilometres and, indirectly, to express the length of the astronomical unit in kilometres. A method now used consists in measuring the time required by an electromagnetic wave (e.g., a radio signal) to make the round trip to the given body and back to Earth. Radar waves and, more recently, laser radiation are used for this purpose. Once the astronomical unit has been calculated by one of these methods, we can express the distance between bodies of the solar system in absolute units (e.g. in kilometres). The diameter D of a planet is found from the formula

$$D = r \sin \varrho \qquad (3\text{-}67)$$

on the basis of the observed angular dimensions ϱ and knowledge of the distance r of that planet from the Earth.

Section 21   Rocket Flights

Rocket flights can be divided into two types:

a) powered flight, in which the rocket engines are operating,

b) inertial or free flight, in which the rocket moves only under the influence of the gravitational attraction of the Earth, Moon, Sun, and planets.

In the first phase of the flight, the rocket motion is due to the action of the engines. During this phase, the rocket attains a predetermined direction and velocity. In subsequent stages of the flight, engines are fired to make corrections in the trajectory, to change the orbit, or to give the rocket some particular spatial orientation. Engines are used in the final phase to brake the rocket so as to bring it back down to Earth.

Jet engines are employed to propel rockets. Combustion products are ejected from a nozzle at a high velocity w (Fig. 3-3). By dm let us denote

Figure 3-3. How a rocket engine functions.

the mass of gas ejected in some interval of time dt. The force required to give this mass a velocity w is

$$P = w \frac{dm}{dt}. \qquad (3\text{-}68)$$

It follows from the third principle of dynamics that a force of the same magnitude, but oppositely directed, acts on the rocket. Thus, the equation of motion for the rocket is

$$m\frac{dv}{dt} = -w\frac{dm}{dt}.$$ (3-69)

From this we have

$$dv = -w\frac{dm}{m}$$ (3-70)

and, upon integration,

$$v = -w\ln m + C.$$ (3-71)

If by M we denote the mass of the rocket at lift-off ($v = 0$), the constant of integration C is

$$C = w\ln M.$$ (3-72)

Insertion of Eq. (3-72) in Eq. (3-71) gives an expression for the velocity attained during powered flight

$$v = w\ln\frac{M}{m}.$$ (3-73)

It is seen from Eq. (73) that the final velocity v of the rocket depends on the velocity w at which the gas is ejected and on the ratio of the masses. The bigger the final mass, the greater the mass of ejected gas $M-m$ must be. The mass m consists of the payload (instrument package), as well as the casing and engines, fuel tanks, etc. As the rocket rises, the amount of fuel decreases and the massive casing required at lift-off becomes superfluous. Thus, an economic way of launching space ships is to use multi-stage rockets. When the fuel has been exhausted in the first stage, the second stage fires and separates from the first, and so on. The last stage serves to put the rocket into a planned orbit.

The discussion above draws attention to the difficulties involved in giving a rocket its initial velocity. It is, therefore, important to calculate the minimum velocity a rocket must have in order to become an artificial satellite of the Earth. For this purpose, we shall show that of all bodies moving in conic sections with the same perigee, a body moving in a circular orbit has the least energy and, hence, the lowest velocity at the perigee.

From Eq. (3-48) we obtain

$$R = \frac{p}{1+e},$$ (3-74)

where R is the distance of the perigee from the centre of the Earth. Since at the perigee the velocity v and the radius vector of the body are perpendicular to each other, by Eqs. (3-41) and (3-33) we have

$$p = \frac{R^2 v^2}{\mu}.$$ (3-75)

It follows from Eqs. (3-74) and (3-75) that the eccentricity e is an increasing linear function of the square of the perigee velocity v:

$$e = \frac{Rv^2}{\mu} - 1.$$ (3-76)

Thus, (since $e \geqslant 0$) the perigee velocity at a given distance from the Earth becomes a minimum when $e = 0$, that is, when the orbit is circular. From Eq. (3-76) we find that this velocity called the first cosmic or circular velocity, is given by the formula

$$v_I = \sqrt{\frac{\mu}{R}} = \sqrt{G\frac{M}{R}},$$ (3-77)

where we have neglected the mass of the rocket in comparison to the Earth's mass M.

A body which has been imparted a velocity $v \geqslant v_I$ at a distance R from the centre of the Earth moves initially along a conic section with perigee at the starting point for inertial flight. Only the gravitational pull of other bodies in the Solar System (chiefly the Moon), and above all the drag of the Earth's atmosphere, can cause the orbital elements to change and, ultimately, to make the satellite fall back to Earth.

In the case of a flight to other planets, we are interested in knowing what minimum velocity a rocket must be given so as to travel in a parabolic or hyperbolic ($e \geqslant 1$) orbit. We see from Eq. (3-76) that this minimum velocity v_{II} will correspond to motion along a parabola ($e = 1$) and is expressed by

$$v_{II} = \sqrt{2\frac{\mu}{R}} = \sqrt{2G\frac{M}{R}}.$$ (3-78)

The velocity v_{II} is called the second cosmic velocity, or parabolic or escape velocity.

For rockets launched from the Earth, $v_I = 7.8$ km/sec and $v_{II} = 11.1$ km/sec. The assumption here is that the perigee of the orbit must be above the dense layers of the atmosphere (hence the assumption $R = 6480$ km).

THE EARTH'S ATMOSPHERE

Research is conducted on the Earth's atmosphere by meteorologists, geophysicists, and astronomers for whom it is a typical planetary atmosphere most accessible to measurements. In recent years, rockets and artificial satellites taking instruments to considerable heights have enabled scientists to make rapid progress in learning the structure of the Earth's atmosphere, especially its upper layers. Measurements in the lower layers, which determine the climate, have long been carried out from ground-based meteorological and geophysical stations and with instruments taken aloft by balloon or aircraft. Further information about the structure of the atmosphere is provided by: analysis of the sunlight which, as it passes through the atmosphere, is absorbed in wavelengths characterizing the chemical composition of the atmosphere; the mode of propagation of sound waves and shock waves produced during explosions above the surface of the Earth; observation of atmospheric effects such as airglow and auroras; the composition and intensity of cosmic radiation observed at various altitudes; the propagation of radio waves, etc.

The purpose of these measurements is to collect information about the pressure, density, temperature, air motion, and chemical composition of the various layers of the atmosphere.

Section 22 General Information

Since the density of the atmosphere decreases rapidly with altitude, most of its mass is concentrated in the layers closest to the Earth. Thus, the chemical composition in the lowest layer of the atmosphere, the troposphere, may be treated as a good approximation of the average chemical composition of the entire atmosphere. Table 3-4 lists the percentage abundance of the principal elements and chemical compounds in the troposphere. In addition to those given in Table 3-4, the air also contains CH_4, H_2, Kr, N_2O, CO, and other constituents.

TABLE 3-4

Chemical Composition of the Troposphere

Constituent	Percentage Abundance by Mass
Nitrogen N_2	78.08
Oxygen O_2	20.95
Argon Ar	0.93
Water vapour H_2O	1–0.001
Carbon dioxide CO_2	0.03
Neon Ne	0.002
Helium He	0.0005

Knowing the sea-level pressure $p(0) = 1013$ mb $= 1.013 \times 10^6$ dyne $\cdot$ cm^{-2}, we can determine the mass of the air contained inside an infinite vertical column 1 cm square. The increment of hydrostatic pressure over a height dh (Cf. Fig. 3-4) is given by the formula

$$dp = -g\varrho dh \qquad (3\text{-}79)$$

or

$$\frac{dp}{dh} = -g\varrho, \qquad (3\text{-}79')$$

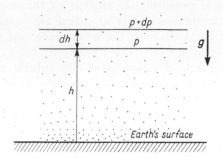

Figure 3-4. Dependence of gasostatic pressure on altitude.

where g is the acceleration due to gravity, and ϱ is the density of the gas at an altitude h. The minus sign on the right-hand side of Eqs. (3-79) and (3-79') indicates that the pressure decreases with altitude h.

Integrating Eq. (3-79') over h from 0 (the surface of the Earth) to ∞ (tentatively we treat the atmosphere as extending infinitely), we obtain

$$\int_0^\infty \frac{dp}{dh}\, dh = -\int_0^\infty g\varrho dh. \tag{3-80}$$

Since the pressure vanishes at the outer edge of the atmosphere (or, in at any event, is much lower than the pressure at the surface of the Earth), the left-hand side of Eq. (3-80) equals

$$p(\infty) - p(0) = -p(0).$$

If we note that the thickness of the layer which contains most of the mass of the atmosphere is small enough for the acceleration due to gravity to be regarded as practically constant and equal to the value at the Earth's surface, we can rewrite the right-hand side of Eq. (3-80) as

$$-\int_0^\infty g\varrho dh = -g\int_0^\infty \varrho dh = -gm,$$

where m is the mass of air lying above 1 cm^2 of the Earth's surface. Hence

$$p(0) = gm, \tag{3-81}$$

from which we have

$$m = \frac{p(0)}{g} = \frac{1.013 \times 10^6}{981}\ \text{g} \cdot \text{cm}^{-2} = 1.033 \times 10^3\ \text{g} \cdot \text{cm}^{-2}. \tag{3-81'}$$

Multiplying this value by the area of the Earth's surface, we obtain $M = 5.25 \times 10^{21}$ g for the mass of the atmosphere. Hence, we see that the mass of the atmosphere constitutes a mere one-millionth of the mass of the Earth.

A homogeneous layer of this mass with the same density as that of the atmosphere at sea level, $\varrho = 1.293 \times 10^{-3}$ g $\cdot$ cm^{-3}, would have a thickness of

$$h = \frac{m}{\varrho} = \frac{1.033 \times 10^3}{1.293 \times 10^{-3}} \text{ cm} \approx 8 \text{ km.} \tag{3-82}$$

Of course, the Earth's atmosphere is not homogeneous; its density decreases with the distance from the surface of the Earth and Eq. (3-82) merely shows that most of the mass of the atmosphere is contained in a layer whose thickness is many times less than the altitude of the Earth's atmosphere as a whole and that extended, much more rarefied layers overlie the lower, high-density layers.

Nor is the atmosphere a uniform medium in regard to chemical composition. Heavier constituents have a tendency to occur in the lower atmosphere (diffusion). On the other hand, turbulent motion, winds, and vertical atmospheric currents tend to reduce the differences in the chemical composition. As a result of these effects in the lower part of the atmosphere, called the homosphere, the chemical composition does not vary much up to an altitude of 80–90 km. Higher up—in the heterosphere—on the other hand, the heavier constituents are seen to become less abundant with altitude (first and foremost, as the altitude increases the percentage abundance of diatomic oxygen and nitrogen decreases while that of monoatomic oxygen and nitrogen rises).

The physical conditions in the atmosphere are determined by the energy flux which flows into it. Since the power of the thermal radiation of the Earth, resulting from the temperature gradient in the Earth's crust, does not exceed 0.03 per cent of the power of solar radiation incident on the upper atmosphere, the Sun may in practice be treated as the sole source of energy in the atmosphere.

The Earth's atmosphere may be heated in several other ways. The upper layers heat up by absorbing short-wave, ultraviolet radiation from the Sun. Radiation which reaches the surface of the Earth determines the thermal conditions in the lower layers. Finally, there is a third way in which solar energy may flow into the atmosphere. The Earth moves through hot interplanetary gas, the extended outer parts of the solar corona (Cf. Secs. 34 and 36). Measurements of the temperature of the upper atmospheric layers show that above 85 km the temperature increases with altitude. No observational data available suggest the existence of a layer, above which the temperature of the atmospheric gas would begin to decrease gradually. This fact evokes the supposition that there is no sharply defined boundary between the atmosphere of the Earth and the interplanetary gas. For the upper limit of the atmosphere we could take that layer which still takes part in the motion of the Earth, i.e. the boundary of the Earth's magnetosphere (for further details see Sec. 28). Since the atmosphere and interplanetary gas are not separated by a sharply-defined boundary, matter and heat must flow between them. Owing to the low heat capacity of the rarefied interplanetary gas, this cannot be decisive in regard to the heat balance of the entire atmosphere but it may be vital in regard to the establishment of a temperature distribution in the upper heterosphere which is also characterized by a low density of matter.

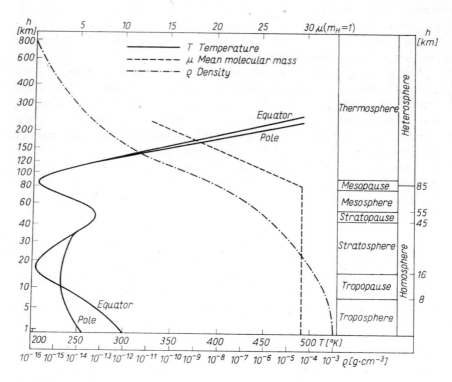

Figure 3-5. Temperature, density, and mean molecular mass in the atmosphere plotted against the altitude above the surface of the Earth.

Thus, the terrestrial atmosphere is a gaseous medium of substantially differentiated physical conditions. It separates into a number of layers which differ from each other in regard to either density, chemical composition, or thermal structure. Each of the layers is characterized by a specific behaviour of the temperature gradient. This is illustrated in Fig. 3-5.

The troposphere, the lowest layer of the atmosphere, stretches from the surface of the Earth to the region known as the tropopause in which the temperature reaches a minimum value of about 200°K. The temperature, which falls off with altitude in the troposphere, again begins to rise above the tropopause—in the stratosphere—to a value of about 270°K at a distance of 50 km above the surface of the Earth. The layer at that altitude, the stratopause, joins the stratosphere to the uppermost layer of the homosphere—the mesosphere, in which the temperature gradient again takes on negative values. The height of these layers is not constant but is subject to seasonal variations and is a function of the geographical latitude. To illustrate these variations in the case of the troposphere let us refer to Fig. 3-6.

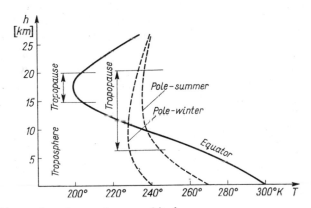

Figure 3-6. Troposphere temperature vs. altitude.

We can see from this figure that the thickness of the troposphere and the extent of the tropopause both depend on the geographical latitude. The tropopause is at a much higher altitude above the equator than it is above the poles. This results in the apparently paradoxical fact that the lowest temperatures in the tropopause occur precisely above the equator whereas the temperature above the poles is about 30 degrees higher.

Section 23   The General Circulation of the Atmosphere
The troposphere plays an important role in distributing heat on the Earth. Since the solar radiation is incident almost vertically, regions of low geographical latitudes receive much more heat than do regions near the poles. On the other hand, calculations indicate that the amount of energy radiated by the surface of the Earth and the surrounding cloud cover does not depend so strongly on the geographical latitude. As a result, equatorial regions receive more energy than they radiate out where as the polar regions lose more heat by radiation than they receive. However,

since—apart from seasonal variations—the mean temperature of the Earth's surface is constant, energy is not stored and the amount of energy received must be equal to the energy loss. Inasmuch as the processes of radiation do not lead to this kind of thermal balance, there must be some other heat flow mechanisms which bring heat to areas of high geographical latitude. The general circulation of the atmosphere is the most efficient process of this kind. Hot air from above the equator rises and forms two currents, one flowing northwards and the other southwards towards the colder regions while cold air flows at a lower level towards the equator.

Superimposed on the motion of these air masses is the deflection caused by Coriolis force. Air masses moving towards the higher geographical latitudes have an excess angular momentum and tend to veer to the East; currents flowing towards the equator veer to the West. Thus, the transport of air masses southwards is accompanied by their motion in the direction of the parallels. If the air masses were to reach the polar regions from the equator without loss of angular momentum (because of, e.g. friction at the Earth's surface and the viscosity of the air), strong winds blowing along the parallels would be observed in the medium geographical latitudes. Since such high-velocity winds are not observed, the supposition that heat is transported along with matter from above the equator to the poles cannot hold. Measurements of the state of the atmosphere and wind velocities have led to the conclusion that the general atmospheric circulation occurs in a different manner in several zones (Cf. Fig. 3-7).

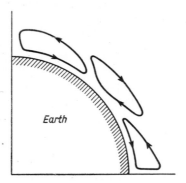

Figure 3-7. General circulation of the atmosphere.

The circulation in the equatorial and circumpolar regions is in accordance with the direction of heat flow in the atmosphere. The fact that the circulation is in the opposite direction in the medium latitudes is explained by the existence of air viscosity.

In our description of circulation we have not made allowance for the local disturbances due to local differences in physical conditions, whereas high or low pressure areas which form above the surface of the Earth are a cause of local motions of air masses. Only when the velocities resulting from the local state of the atmosphere are superimposed upon the general circulation of the air do we obtain the distribution of winds in the atmosphere as observed by the meteorologists.

Section 24 The Chemical Composition of the Atmosphere

Table 3-4 gives the chemical composition of the troposphere. We said earlier that this composition is approximately the same throughout the entire homosphere. This is true primarily in regard to the most abundant constituents. However, the optical properties of the atmosphere depend strongly on less abundant constituents such as ozone, water vapour, and carbon dioxide which have strong absorption bands in that part of the electromagnetic spectrum in which solar radiation occurs.

Carbon dioxide comes into being, among other ways, as the result of biochemical processes at the Earth's surface from which it is carried upwards. Measurements have not revealed any major differences in the percentage abundance of carbon dioxide to a height of several tens of kilometres.

The amount of water vapour in the lower atmosphere is subject to pronounced seasonal variations and depends on the meteorological conditions in the area under study. Measurements of humidity with balloon-borne hygrometers show that the water vapour content in the stratosphere is about 0.004 per cent. Other types of measurements of the water vapour content in the atmosphere are based on observations of the absorption bands in the spectrum of sunlight. Water vapour absorbs a number of narrow bands in the 1–3 μ range, a very strong and wide band about 6.3 μ, and a broad band starting from about 20 μ and extending into the long-wavelength region of the spectrum. Observations of the intensity of these bands in the solar spectrum enables us to establish the amount of water vapour present in the layers of the atmosphere traversed by the radiation. If the absorption bands are measured at various altitudes, the vertical distribution of the water vapour in the atmosphere can be determined.

Short-wave solar radiation causes oxygen molecules to dissociate. Diatomic molecules of oxygen O_2, which have a dissociation energy of 5.2 eV, intensively absorb quanta of higher energy ($\lambda < 2400$ Å) to split into two atoms of oxygen O

$$O_2 + h\nu \rightarrow O + O, \quad h\nu > 5.2 \text{ eV}. \tag{3-83}$$

The single atoms of oxygen combine with diatomic molecules of oxygen to form molecules of ozone. Since two molecules (an O_2 molecule and an O atom) form a single molecule of ozone during this reaction, some other molecule M of the medium must act as a catalyst in order for the energy and momentum of the components taking part in the reaction to be conserved. Consequently, the ozone-production reaction is written as

$$O_2 + O + M \rightarrow O_3 + M. \tag{3-84}$$

The ozone molecules, which are less stable than those of diatomic oxygen, dissociate under the influence of radiation of wavelength $\lambda < 11,000$ Å

$$O_3 + h\nu \rightarrow O_2 + O, \quad h\nu > 1.1 \text{ eV}. \tag{3-85}$$

Ozone can also be converted into diatomic oxygen in the reaction

$$O_3 + O \rightarrow 2O_2. \tag{3-86}$$

The rate of reactions (3-83) and (3-85) in this cycle depends on the intensity and spectral distribution of the radiation, while the rate of reactions (3-84) and (3-86) depends on the frequency of collisions of gas molecules. Thus, the conditions at different altitudes are conducive to one reaction or another. This explains the nonuniform distribution of various forms of oxygen in the atmosphere. In the upper layers, where the intensity of the ionizing radiation is high, reaction (3-83) leads to the formation of monoatomic oxygen. Owing to the low density of the medium, molecules rarely collide and, consequently, the probability of their recombining into a di- or triatomic molecule is small. Reaction (3-84) can take place in the lower, denser layers, where ozone is observed to occur. The ozone molecules photodissociate [reaction (3-85)], or interact with oxygen atoms [reaction (3-86)], to break down into di- or monoatomic molecules of oxygen. Finally, in the lowest layer, which is not reached by any radiation of wavelength $\lambda < 2400$ Å, no dissociation of oxygen molecules occurs. Forms of oxygen produced at various altitudes are partly transported to adjoining layers by diffusion and by the convection of air masses. These phenomena are also responsible for the presence of ozone in the troposphere.

As a result of these processes, a layer of maximum ozone concentration, the ozonosphere, is formed in the stratosphere. The percentage abundance of monoatomic oxygen, on the other hand, increases with altitude so that in the heterosphere, starting from an altitude of about 120 km, it exceeds the content of molecular oxygen.

Ozone strongly absorbs radiation in a band about 2600 Å (the Hartley band). Absorption in this band prevents ultraviolet radiation with a wavelength of $\lambda < 3000$ Å from reaching the surface of the Earth. The absorption of radiation heats up the air, causing the temperature to rise with altitude in the stratosphere. In addition to absorption in the ultraviolet, ozone also absorbs a weaker band about $\lambda = 5700$ Å (Chappius band)

and bands in the infrared with wavelength of about 5, 9.6, and 14 μ. The position of the ozonosphere and its ozone content have been studied by several methods, chiefly spectroscopy.

Let us consider how the amount of transmitted light I_λ at some wavelength λ depends on the thickness x of the ozone layer traversed by that radiation. Imagine that we isolate an ozone layer of thickness ds (Fig. 3-8). The decrease of radiation intensity in this layer, $-dI_\lambda$, is proportional to the amount of incident radiation

$$- dI_\lambda = a_\lambda I_\lambda, \tag{3-87}$$

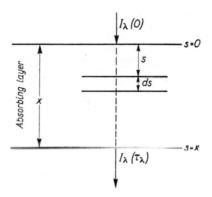

Figure 3-8. The absorption of radiation in the absorbing layer.

where the coefficient a_λ is proportional to the thickness ds of the layer and the density ϱ and also depends on the optical properties of the medium for the given wavelength. The value of a for a 1-cm layer in which the density is 1 g·cm^{-3} is called the coefficient of absorption for the given gas and is denoted by $\varkappa_\lambda$. Therefore, for a layer of density ϱ and thickness ds, this ceofficient is

$$a_\lambda = \varkappa_\lambda \varrho ds. \tag{3-88}$$

Thus, Eq. (3-87) can be rewritten as

$$-dI_\lambda = \varkappa_\lambda \varrho I_\lambda ds \tag{3-89}$$

or

$$\frac{dI_\lambda}{I_\lambda} = -\varkappa_\lambda \varrho ds. \tag{3-90}$$

Integration of Eq. (3-90) over ds from 0 to x yields

$$\ln I_\lambda \Big|_0^x = -\int_0^x \varkappa_\lambda \varrho ds. \tag{3-91}$$

The value of $\int_{0}^{x} \varkappa_\lambda \varrho\, ds$ is called the optical thickness of the medium and is denoted by τ_λ. Thus, by Eq. (3-91) we have

$$I_\lambda(\tau_\lambda) = I_\lambda(0)e^{-\tau_\lambda}, \tag{3-92}$$

where $I_\lambda(\tau_\lambda)$ is the intensity the radiation has upon travelling through the medium over a distance equal to the optical thickness τ_λ.

Equation (3-92) leads to the statement:

The intensity of radiation passing through an absorbent medium decreases exponentially with the optical thickness of the medium.

An analogous statement can be made in reference to the case of a scattering medium.

Measuring the intensity of the ozone absorption lines in solar radiation spectra obtained at various altitudes above the Earth's surface (Plate 5), we can find the optical thickness of overlying layers by using Eq. (3-92). Then we can determine the density of ozone as a function of the altitude (the coefficient of absorption $\varkappa_\lambda$ is known from measurements in the laboratory).

In Figures (3-9) and (3-10) the ozone content in the atmosphere is plotted against the altitude above sea level. These figures show, for instance, that even in the layer of maximum content (about 25–30 km above sea level) ozone constitutes less than one one-hundred-thousandth of the mass of the air.

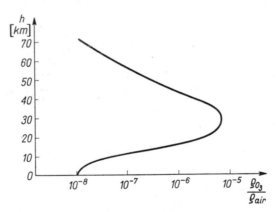

Figure 3-9. Ozone-to-air density ratio vs. altitude.

Other molecules also dissociate under the influence of ultraviolet radiation. Water vapour breaks down into hydrogen H and hydroxide OH. Carbon dioxide CO_2 dissociates into atomic oxygen O and carbon dioxide CO. Just as oxygen, nitrogen occurs in atomic form in the higher layers

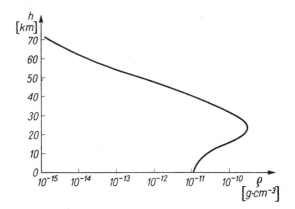

Figure 3-10. Ozone density plotted against the altitude above the Earth.

of the atmosphere. The presence of active ions and atoms leads to a number of chemical reactions. Energy first absorbed in the dissociation processes is then emitted as a result of chemical reactions, causing the atmosphere to glow.

Section 25   The Heat Balance of the Homosphere

The distribution of radiation intensity in the solar spectrum can be described with great accuracy by Planck's formula

$$I_\lambda = c_1 \lambda^{-5} \left[e^{\frac{c_2}{\lambda k T}} - 1 \right]^{-1}, \tag{3-93}$$

where c_1 and c_2 are constants, $k = 1.381 \times 10^{-16}$ erg $\cdot$ deg^{-1} is Boltzmann's constant, and T denotes the temperature of the solar photosphere (about 6000°K). Solar radiation has its maximum intensity at a wavelength of about 5000 Å. Almost the entire energy emitted by the Sun is contained in the spectral region from 1500 Å in the ultraviolet to 50,000 Å in the infrared (Cf. Fig. 3-11a).

Assumption of Eq. (3-93) as an approximation of the spectral distribution of the solar radiation corresponds to the assumption that the photosphere of the Sun may be treated as an ideal black body. Further details about the spectrum of solar radiation will be given in the next chapter. For the time being we shall confine ourselves to pointing out the two principal ways in which the distribution of the solar radiation spectrum deviates from the distribution given by Planck's formula:

1. Spectroscopic observations made from rockets above the ozonosphere reveal a distinct deficit of ultraviolet radiation as compared to Eq. (3-93).

2. The spectrum as specified by Planck's formula is continuous whereas in the actual spectrum of the Sun we observe a number of absorption

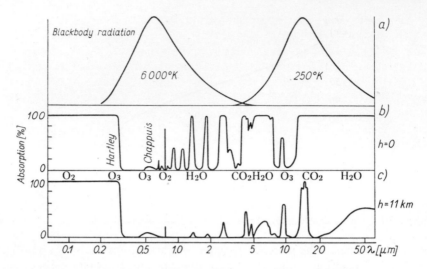

Figure 3-11. a) Blackbody emission at 6000°K and 250°K; b) absorption of radiation upon traversing layers above 11 km. [After Goody and Robinson, *Quarterly Journ. Roy. Meteorogical Soc.* **75**, 161 (1951)].

lines (Fraunhofer lines) caused by absorption in the atmosphere of the Sun.

Solar radiation is absorbed as it passes through the Earth's atmosphere. The far ultraviolet part of the spectrum is partly absorbed by oxygen and nitrogen molecules in the heterosphere. The stratosphere is heated mainly by radiation absorbed strongly by ozone in the Hartley band at an altitude of 30 to 50 km. Finally, in the troposphere, water vapour absorbs a number of bands in the infrared. The result is that part of the solar radiation is absorbed in the atmosphere. The spectral distribution of this radiation, whose energy is used (generally speaking) to heat the atmosphere, is obtained if the intensity of the radiation arriving from the Sun as a function of the wavelength (the curve for 6000°K in Fig. 3-11a) is multiplied by the value of the atmospheric absorption (Fig. 3-11b). The rest of the radiation, with the spectral distribution now different than that of the Sun's, reaches the surface of the Earth where part is absorbed by the soil and part is reflected.

This flux of energy flowing downwards is accompanied by another, directed upwards, produced by the thermal radiation from the Sun-heated Earth and its atmosphere. The energy contained in both of these fluxes (apart from instantaneous variations of temperature) must be the same. Since it is impossible for large quantities of heat to be stored on the Earth and in the atmosphere, the amount of energy received from the Sun must equal the amount of energy radiated out.

The Earth and the troposphere emit radiation corresponding approximately to the radiation of a body at a temperature of about 250°K (Fig. 3-11a). This region of the spectrum, between 6 μ and 60 μ, contains many intense bands, especially those of water vapour as well as those of carbon dioxide, nitrogen oxide, and ozone. In the case of a dense cloud cover, the thermal radiation of the Earth is absorbed strongly at low altitudes; as a result, radiation of heat from the surface of the Earth is hindered and the temperature in the area under consideration (at night, when the given area is not receiving energy from the Sun) is higher than it would be under similar conditions but with a cloudless sky. Thermal radiation is emitted from the atmosphere in the same bands in which atmospheric absorption occurs. Superposition of the second curve (250°K) from Fig. 3-11a and the curve from Fig. 3-11c yields the spectral distribution of the thermal radiation of the Earth's atmosphere.

The picture of the thermal relations of our atmosphere would not be complete if it were not emphasized that energy transfer by convection, especially in the troposphere, is highly important for the vertical and horizontal distribution of temperature. Only if all the possible modes of energy transfer—radiation, convection, as well as thermal conduction in some layers—are taken into account can one understand the observed temperature distribution in the atmosphere.

Section 26   The Ionosphere

Solar radiation causes partial ionization of molecules (from an altitude of about 50–60 km and higher) throughout the entire heterosphere. This is why the gas present in the heterosphere is a mixture of ions, electrons, and neutral particles. Collisions between ions and electrons lead to their recombining into neutral molecules. As a result of these interactions, the number of electrons per unit volume is constant when the rates of photoionization processes (producing ions) and recombination processes (reducing their number) are equal. We then say that ionization equilibrium is established in the medium. However, since the rate of these processes is not the same at all altitudes, characteristic layers with various ion contents form in the atmosphere. That part of the atmosphere in which free electrons and ions occur is called the ionosphere, and its consecutive layers with maximum electron (and ion) content are denoted by the letters D, E, F.

Let us now consider on what the rate of the ionization and recombination processes depends. Ionizing solar radiation incident from above reaches deeper- and deeper-lying layers of the atmosphere. On the way, it encounters an increasing number of ionizable molecules and neutral atoms in each cubic centimetre. Thus, the number of ionization events, and hence the number of ions produced and electrons freed, increases with the depth. At the same time, this radiation is also absorbed since the energy it carries is lost during ionization in order to overcome the forces binding the electrons in the shells of the molecules. Thus, with increasing optical depth the number of quanta capable of causing ionization is reduced and the number of electrons produced begins to fall off from a certain altitude. In this way, a layer in which the process of ionization is most efficient is formed in the atmosphere and above and below it fewer ions are produced per unit time and volume.

The number $\mathscr{I}$ of free electrons coming into being per second per cm^3 as a result of photoionization can be expressed by the formula

$$\mathscr{I} = aIn(A), \tag{3-94}$$

where I is the ionizing radiation intensity which decreases with depth, $n(A)$ is the density of ionizable molecules, and a is a proportionality factor.

Free electrons are lost in several ways, the most effective in the atmosphere being:

a) recombination coupled with simultaneous radiation of a quantum of energy;

b) binding of electrons with neutral atoms or molecules into negative ions;

c) recombination with the participation of a neutral molecule.

a) The loss of electrons owing to direct recombination

$$A^+ + e^- \rightarrow A + h\nu \tag{3-95}$$

(where A^+ denotes a positive ion, e^- an electron, A the resultant neutral atom, and $h\nu$ is the energy radiated during the recombination) is proportional to the electron density $n(e^-)$ and positive ion density $n(A^+)$ in the region under consideration. If by $\mathscr{R}$ we denote the number of recombination events per cm^3 per second, then

$$\mathscr{R} = \alpha n(A^+)n(e^-), \tag{3-96}$$

where the proportionality factor α is called the recombination coefficient.

In regions where the number of negative ions is low, the number of electrons must be approximately equal to the number of positive ions

$$n(A^+) = n(e^-). \tag{3-97}$$

Otherwise, the region in question would have an excess charge of one sign (positive or negative) which would result in electric currents that would transport charge to adjoining regions until Eq. (3-97) were satisfied. If Eq. (3-97) is taken into account, Eq. (3-96) can be rewritten as

$$\mathscr{R} = \alpha n^2(e^-). \tag{3-98}$$

Ionization equilibrium occurs when the number of electrons produced by photoionization is equal to the number of recombinations, that is, when

$$\mathcal{J} = \mathcal{R}. \tag{3-99}$$

Thus, in regions where the loss of free electrons is due primarily to direct recombination with positive ions, the electron density—as emerges from Eqs. (3-94), (3-98), and (3-99)—is expressed by the formula

$$n(e^-) = \sqrt{\frac{aIn(A)}{\alpha}} = \sqrt{\frac{\mathcal{J}}{\alpha}} \tag{3-100}$$

that is, is proportional to the square root of the intensity and the density.

b) Oxygen atoms and molecules play the main role in the formation of negative ions in the atmosphere. The reactions

$$O_2 + e^- \rightarrow O_2^- + h\nu \tag{3-101}$$

and

$$O + e^- \rightarrow O^- + h\nu \tag{3-102}$$

lead to the formation of negative ions of oxygen. The loss of free electrons is in this case proportional to the density of oxygen atoms and molecules and to the electron density

$$\mathcal{R} = \beta_1 n(e^-)n(O_2) + \beta_2 n(e^-)n(O) = [\beta_1 n(O_2) + \beta_2 n(O)]n(e^-). \tag{3-103}$$

Negative ions recombining with positive ions form neutral particles. Since the degree of ionization in regions where negative ions are produced is in general small, i.e.

$$n(O_2) \gg n(e^-) \tag{3-104}$$

and

$$n(O) \gg n(e^-) \tag{3-105}$$

the number of neutral molecules per cm^3 practically does not depend on how many molecules have been ionized or negative ions produced; that is to say, the expression

$$\beta_1 n(O_2) + \beta_2 n(O) = \beta(\varrho) \tag{3-106}$$

does not depend on the degree of ionization but only on the gas density ϱ. Therefore, Eq. (3-103) can be rewritten in the form

$$\mathcal{R} = \beta(\varrho)n(e^-). \tag{3-107}$$

Thus, the number of free electrons in layers in which they are lost primarily by being bound into negative ions, is given by the formula

$$n(e^-) = \frac{\alpha In(A)}{\beta(\varrho)} = \frac{\mathcal{J}}{\beta(\varrho)}. \tag{3-108}$$

c) The third way in which electrons are lost in the ionosphere is through the following cycle of reactions:

$$O^+ + O_2 \rightarrow O_2^+ + O, \tag{3-109}$$

$$O_2^+ + e^- \rightarrow O + O. \tag{3-110}$$

A charge exchange between an ionized atom of oxygen and a neutral diatomic molecule of oxygen—reaction (3-109)—is followed by recombination of the electron with simultaneous dissociation into two oxygen atoms— reaction (3-110). If the number of ions of diatomic oxygen is to be constant, the number of events in which reaction (3-109) occurs must be equal to the number of events in which reaction (3-110) takes place. On the other hand, ionization equilibrium is attained when the number of atoms recombining during reaction (3-110) equals the number of photoionization events $\mathcal{J}$. Therefore

$$\gamma_1 n(O^+) n(O_2) = \gamma_2 n(O_2^+) n(e^-) = \mathcal{J}, \tag{3-111}$$

where γ_1 and γ_2 are proportionality factors.

This equation yields the number of positive ions of monoatomic and diatomic oxygen:

$$n(O^+) = \frac{\mathcal{J}}{\gamma_1 n(O_2)} \tag{3-112}$$

and

$$n(O_2^+) = \frac{\mathcal{J}}{\gamma_2 n(e^-)}. \tag{3-113}$$

At the same time, the number of molecules of negative electric charge must be equal to the number of molecules of positive charge. Hence,

$$n(e^-) = n(O^+) + n(O_2^+) \tag{3-114}$$

or

$$n(e^-) = \frac{\mathcal{J}}{\gamma_1 n(O_2)} + \frac{\mathcal{J}}{\gamma_2 n(e^-)} \tag{3-115}$$

and therefore

$$\mathcal{J} = \frac{\gamma_1 \gamma_2 n(O_2)}{\gamma_1 n(O_2) + \gamma_2 n(e^-)} n^2(e^-). \tag{3-116}$$

In addition to the electron density $n(e^-)$ and the number of photoionization events $\mathcal{J}$, Eq. (3-116) also contains a third variable: the oxygen molecule density $n(O_2)$ which decreases with altitude. Up to an altitude of about 200 km, where the density of oxygen molecules is still sufficiently high, we can neglect $\gamma_2 n(e^-)$ in comparison with $\gamma_1 n(O_2)$, and Eq. (3-116) can be rewritten as

$$\mathcal{J} \approx \gamma_2 n^2(e^-). \tag{3-117}$$

In this area the electron density is given by a formula analogous to Eq. (3-110). However, in layers more than 200 km above the Earth's surface, the density of oxygen molecules is much lower. Then

$$\gamma_1 n(O_2) \ll \gamma_2 n(e^-) \qquad (3\text{-}118)$$

and Eq. (3-116) becomes

$$\mathscr{I} \approx \gamma_1 n(O_2) n(e^-) \qquad (3\text{-}119)$$

or

$$n(e^-) \approx \frac{\mathscr{I}}{\gamma_1 n(O_2)}. \qquad (3\text{-}120)$$

As in Eq. (3-108), a gas density increasing with altitude appears in the denominator of Eq. (3-120). For illustration, reactions (b) and (c) have been discussed here as reactions with oxygen atoms and molecules. Similar reactions may, however, also occur with the participation of other elements, above all nitrogen.

Knowing the rate $\mathscr{I}$ at which they are produced, we can determine the density $n(e^-)$ of free electrons at any point in the ionosphere from Eqs. (3-100), (3-108), and (3-116). The choice of formula depends on the conditions in the given layer, on the pressure, temperature, density of matter, and chemical composition. In practice, it proves insufficient in general to use only one of these equations—(3-100), (3-108) or (3-116)—to find the electron density. Instead, a combination of them is employed since electrons may be lost not only in one way but simultaneously in two or all three ways listed in points (a), (b), and (c).

Note an interesting property that Eqs. (3-100) and (3-117) have: $n(e^-)$ found from these formulae is a monotone function of $\mathscr{I}$. Thus, the layer of maximum electron density, defined by the equation

$$\frac{dn(e^-)}{dh} = 0 \qquad (3\text{-}121)$$

(where h is the altitude above the Earth's surface), comes at the place where

$$\frac{d\mathscr{I}}{dh} = 0 \qquad (3\text{-}122)$$

which means that this layer is exactly where the production of electrons is greatest.

The situation is different in regions where Eqs. (3-108) and (3-120) hold. The maximum electron density depends here not only on the electron production rate but also on the atmospheric density, which varies with altitude. Since $n(O)$ and $n(O_2)$ in the denominator decrease, the electron density increases with altitude and the maximum does not occur in the layer of greatest electron production, but higher up. This is most probably why the uppermost layer of the ionosphere, the F layer, splits into two: the F_1 layer at an altitude of about 170 km, and a very thick F_2 layer above 200 km.

At the beginning of this section we discussed the ionizing radiation in general terms, without specifying its spectrum. As it passes through the ionosphere, this radiation is absorbed in different fashion for various wavelengths and, consequently, the spectrum of this radiation changes. At the same time, this radiation reaches layers of ever different chemical composition—the ionizable constituents change with the depth in the atmosphere. This is precisely why there are several ionospheric layers D, E, F, and not just one.

Strong absorption of radiation of wavelengths shorter than 900 Å by oxygen and nitrogen is responsible for photoionization in the F layer; X radiation shorter than 100 Å reaches deeper, causing the E layer to be formed at an altitude of about 100 km. Radiation with a wavelength of about 1200 Å, which is absorbed to a lesser extent in oxygen and nitrogen, gets down to at an altitude of 70 km, where the D layer comes into being, probably as a result of the ionization of nitrogen oxide (Cf. Fig. 3-12).

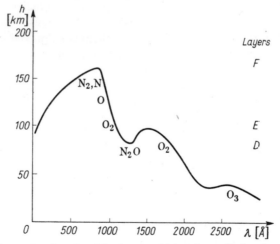

Figure 3-12. Curve showing the altitudes at which solar radiation is attenuated by a factor of e. The symbols denote the most active absorbers.

Studies of the propagation of radio waves in the ionosphere constitute a major source of information about the ionosphere. Electromagnetic waves are subject to refraction and reflection in ionized media. The frequency of radiation which undergoes reflection depends on the electron density. A medium of higher electron density is capable of reflecting waves with higher frequencies. This fact is used to determine the degree of ionization in the atmosphere. Measurement of the time a signal takes to travel to an ionospheric layer and be bounced back to the receiver after reflection serves to establish the altitude of the layer under study. In recent years, rockets have been used to emit or receive radio waves right in the iono-sphere. The results of these measurements, plotted on a diagram called an ionogram (Cf. Fig. 3-13), provide a basis for investigating the vertical distribution of the electron density in the ionosphere (Fig. 3-14). Measure-

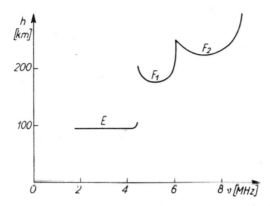

Figure 3-13. An example of an ionogram. A diagram of the altitudes at which radio waves of a given frequency are reflected.

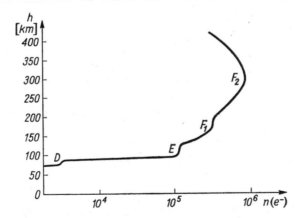

Figure 3-14. Electron density vs. altitude.

ments with rocket-borne mass spectrometers have led to the direct detection in the ionosphere of O_2^+, O^+, NO^+, N_2^+, N^+ and other positive ions as well as the negative ions NO_2^-, O_2^-, and O^-.

The state of the ionosphere, the electron density, depends in great measure on the solar illumination at various times in the day, the solar activity, and the intensity of the flux of cosmic radiation. Both the altitude at which electrons occur, and their density, in the ionospheric layers are subject to large periodic variations.

Section 27   The Earth's Magnetic Field

We can distinguish two components of the Earth's magnetic field: 1) a regular field which is approximately constant in time, 2) a less intense, rapidly-varying field due to electromagnetic phenomena occurring in the atmosphere.

1. The regular magnetic field of the Earth may be approximated with a considerable degree of accuracy by the field of a dipole placed in the interior of the Earth (Fig. 3-15). The points on the Earth's surface at which

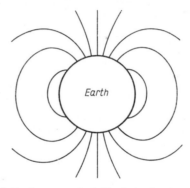

Figure 3-15. Diagram of dipole magnetic field of the Earth.

the magnetic field lines are perpendicular to that surface are known as the magnetic poles of the Earth. The straight line passing through the poles is called the Earth's magnetic axis. The magnetic axis is inclined to the axis of rotation and does not pass through the centre of the Earth; the positions of the magnetic poles are: 73° 30′ north latitude, 92° 30′ west longitude, and 72° 25′ south latitude, and 154° east longitude.

2. The ebbs and tides in the Earth's atmosphere, due to the attraction of the Sun and the Moon, differences in pressure, and other factors, are the cause of strong ionospheric winds. Electric currents are produced in partially (or totally) ionized gas moving in a magnetic field just as in a conductor. These currents are perpendicular to the direction of the magnetic field and the velocity of the gas. The wind speed in the E layer can be as high as 100 m/sec. Electric currents arise in the E layer as a result of this motion of the gas with respect to the magnetic field. This phenomenon is called the "atmospheric dynamo". The currents induced in turn generate

magnetic fields which, being superimposed on the regular component, are detected at the Earth's surface as variations in the direction and intensity of the general magnetic field. The magnetic fields induced in the E layer also get into the upper layers of the atmosphere and cause electric currents in the F layer. When electric currents flow through a gas in a magnetic field, the gas is acted upon by a Lorentz force perpendicular to the direction of the current and of the magnetic field. This force is probably responsible for the vertical motions of the F layer. This phenomenon is known as the "atmospheric motor".

Section 28   Incident Cosmic Radiation and the Magnetosphere

Back in the Twenties it was observed that the intensity of cosmic radiation at the surface of the Earth depends on the geomagnetic latitude at the place of measurement. The intensity of this radiation is higher in the proximity of the magnetic poles than near the equator. This fact indicates that charged particles are present in primary cosmic radiation. Further investigation showed that primary cosmic radiation consists primarily of the nuclei—stripped of their electron shells—of hydrogen (83–89% protons), as well as helium (10–15% alpha particles), and slight amounts (1–2%) of heavier elements, chiefly oxygen, carbon, boron, magnesium, silicon, nitrogen, and iron. Primary cosmic radiation is also made up of neutrons, electrons, and gamma rays. The intensity of primary cosmic radiation varies somewhat (in general not exceeding 10% of the total intensity) owing mainly to the presence of active centres on the Sun (Cf. Sec. 37). Nevertheless, when averaged over longer periods of time this intensity (especially that of high-energy particles) does not display any major variations. A very important feature of cosmic radiation is that it is isotropic beyond the Earth's atmosphere. Both these facts are evidence that cosmic radiation does not originate from a principal source associated with some body in the Solar System but comes from interstellar space.

When particles of primary cosmic radiation collide with nuclei of atoms in the atmosphere, the latter disintegrate and the ensuing secondary radiation causes a cascade of particles, the last stage of which reaches the Earth. Thus, the composition of the cosmic radiation observed at the Earth's surface (mesons, protons, neutrons, electrons, and gamma rays) differs substantially from the composition of the primary radiation.

One of the greatest geophysical discoveries in recent years was Van Allen's identification of two belts of radiation around the Earth on the basis of measurements made by instruments on board Explorer I and Explorer II in 1958. These belts occur above the geomagnetic equator at altitudes of about 3000–4000 km and 15,000–25,000 km (Fig. 3-16).

The inner Van Allen belt contains protons posseessing energies of the order of 100 Mev and electrons with energies of up to about 1 Mev. The

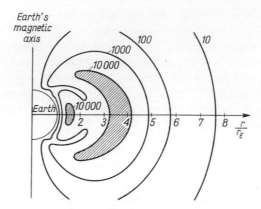

Figure 3-16. Radiation belts. The figures denote the number of particles recorded in a second by a Geiger counter. The distance is expressed in Earth radii.

position of this belt does not change much with time. The outer belt, which varies much more in height, contains protons with energies of tens of Mev and electrons whose energy does not exceed 100 kev.

In principle, there may be two sources of the particles occurring in the Van Allen belts. One is the influx of ionized gas from the solar corona. The other is that of corpuscular radiation of the atmosphere induced by cosmic radiation. Some of the neutrons produced during the disintegration of nuclei bombarded by cosmic radiation in the atmosphere move upwards. The stream of these neutrons, which are electrically neutral particles, can move without perturbations from the magnetic field to considerable heights above the surface of the Earth. There the neutrons decay (the mean lifetime of a neutron is 900 seconds) into protons, electrons, and neutrinos. Neutrinos leave the environs of the Earth, whereas the magnetic field halts further vertical motion of the protons and electrons.

The protons and electrons "populating" the radiation belts can spiral about the magnetic field lines. At greater geomagnetic latitudes, where the field lines approach each other (the intensity of the field increases) the spiral becomes tighter and tighter, and in the end the particle undergoes reflection, changing the direction of its motion. Such a particle is caught in a "magnetic trap" (particle B in Fig. 3-17). On the other hand, particles which move almost exactly along the magnetic field lines can penetrate into the atmosphere (particle A in Fig. 3-17) in the polar regions where the lines of magnetic force are directed towards the Earth's surface. At altitudes of about 200–300 km, they make the temperature rise in the proximity of the poles (Cf. Fig. 3-5) and are one of the causes of the auroras.

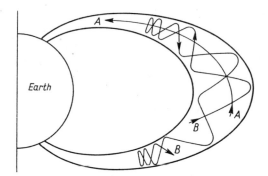

Figure 3-17. Trajectories of particles in the terrestrial magnetic field.

That part of the space around the Earth where ionized matter moves under the action of the terrestrial magnetic field is called the Earth's magnetosphere. It encompasses the entire atmosphere, the Van Allen belts are contained within it, and the shape of its outer surface is determined by the interaction of the interplanetary medium. Whereas adoption of a dipole field was a good approximation of the actual structure of the magnetic

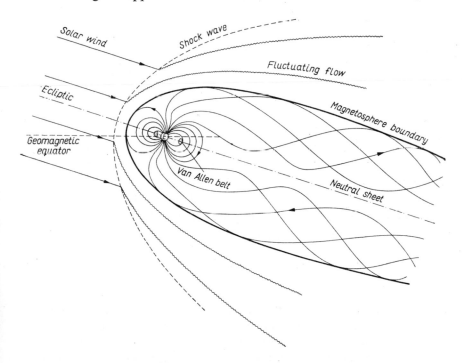

Figure 3-18. Shape of the field lines in the Earth's magnetosphere.

field in the inner magnetosphere, this approximation is not correct in parts more distant from the Earth. The Earth's magnetosphere is a sort of obstacle to the stream of matter, called the solar wind (Cf. Sec. 33), flowing from the Sun. The solar wind strikes the part of the magnetosphere facing the Sun at supersonic speeds producing a shock wave (known as bow shock) at its boundary and then flows around the whole magnetosphere. In effect, the symmetry of the magnetosphere is perturbed. In the forward part facing the Sun, its boundary (delineated by a balance between the external pressure due to the momentum of the solar wind particles and the internal pressure due to the terrestrial magnetic field in this region) lies about 64,000 km from the centre of the Earth; in the opposite direction, the magnetosphere stretches out to considerable distances. The lines of force of the magnetic field coming out of regions lying very close to the poles, are blown by the solar wind and directed in the anti-solar direction. Because of the rotation of the Earth, they are twisted into two convolutions of opposite polarity on either side of the plane of the Earth's equator. (Cf. Fig. 3-18).

PLANETARY ATMOSPHERES AND INTERPLANETARY MATTER

Using the Earth's atmosphere as an example, we have tried to follow the main physical phenomena typical of the atmospheres of planets. The state of a planetary atmosphere depends in the first place on 1) its mass, 2) its chemical composition, 3) the intensity of the solar radiation falling on it or the temperature of the planet, and 4) the acceleration due to gravity at the surface of the planet. Knowledge of these elements is sufficient to enable us to build a schematic model of the atmosphere. Thus, we shall confine ourselves to a cursory survey of the properties of planetary atmospheres, as listed in points (1)–(4), and especially their chemical composition.

Section 29   Mercury

The temperature of Mercury (Plate 6) is about 600°K. Since the acceleration due to gravity at Mercury's surface is low (the planet has a small mass), gas molecules above its surface easily acquire parabolic velocities sufficient to escape from the planet. For this reason Mercury's atmosphere, if it were to exist, would quickly be diffused. This is confirmed by observations; no atmosphere has been detected in many attempts made thus far. A weak effect, which could be interpreted as an argument for the existence of an atmosphere, occurs in measurements of the polarization of Mercury's disk. The amount of gas per cm^2 planetary surface determined in this way is less than 1/300th of the Earth's atmosphere. It is difficult to say whether this estimate is realistic, since this effect may be equally explained without assuming the existence of an atmosphere on Mercury.

Section 30   Venus

In contrast to Mercury, Venus (Plate 7) is characterized by a dense, extended atmosphere. The clouds enveloping the planet prevent observation of the lower layers of the atmosphere and of the surface of the planet itself. For this reason, the rotation period of Venus. (243.16 days) has been estimated from radar measurements but a few years ago. An important source of information about the Venusian atmosphere is that of measurements of thermal radio emission at millimetre and centimetre wavelengths since thermal radiation can come from deeper layers of the atmosphere than can optical radiation. Inasmuch as the intensity of this radiation depends on the temperature of the emitting layers, we thus gain information about the temperature distribution in the atmosphere of Venus.

Temperatures determined from observations in the region of wavelengths of several centimetres are about 580°K, whereas in shorter waves they are only 300–400°K as can be seen in Table 3-5. This difference may indicate

TABLE 3-5

Temperature of Venusian Atmosphere From Radio
Measurements

Wavelength (cm)	Temperature (°K)	Wavelength (cm)	Temperature (°K)
0.80	315	3.4	575
0.86	410	3.75	585
3.15	595	9.4	580
3.37	575	10.2	600

that the radiation in the 0.80–0.86-cm interval comes from the upper layers of the atmosphere, whereas radiation with a wavelength of several centimetres comes from much deeper, hotter layers, and perhaps from the very surface of the planet.

The arrival of centimetre radio radiation from deep layers of the atmosphere can be explained only by a low content of water vapour and oxygen, constituents which are highly absorbed in this part of the spectrum. Carbon dioxide CO_2, which has also been detected by spectroscopic studies of optical radiation, strongly absorbs millimetre waves, the result being that radiation at these wavelengths reaches us only from the outer layers of the atmosphere.

The temperature, pressure, and chemical composition of the Venusian atmosphere have been measured directly by instruments carried by the space probes Venus 4 (October 1967), and Venus 5 and Venus 6 (May 1969). These probes did not reach the surface of the planet since they were crushed by the extremely high pressure of the atmosphere, probably several tens or more than a hundred times the atmospheric pressure on the Earth's surface. It has been found that the atmosphere of Venus consists almost wholly of carbon dioxide; oxygen and water vapour constitute about 1.5% of the total mass of the atmosphere and no detectable traces of nitrogen were found. Nor was the presence of a magnetic field and radiation belts around the planet observed.

Section 31   Mars

So-called polar caps which form alternately around the poles of Mars are obvious features on the disk of the planet (Plate 8). The seasonal appearance of the polar caps, the formation and disappearance of clouds, and the occurrence of a misty halo around the planet in blue light testify to the existence of an atmosphere on Mars. The spectrum of light reflected from the polar caps is identical with the spectrum of light reflected from ice. This is evidence that water exists on Mars, despite the lack of spectroscopic confirmation of the presence of water vapour in the atmosphere. Similarly, the oxygen content is at least one thousand times lower in the Martian atmosphere than in the Earth's atmosphere. On the other hand, the amount of carbon dioxide per cm^2 of planetary surface is probably about 13 times greater on Mars.

The surface of Mars was inspected from a distance of several thousand kilometres by Mariner 4 in July 1965 and Mariners 6 and 7 in July 1969. Photographs taken of the planet's surface have revealed the existence of a large number of meteorite craters on Mars (Plate 9). Measurements of the atmospheric density have led to the conclusion that the pressure at the surface of Mars does not exceed several millibars, or about one-tenth the value found from previous investigations. No appreciable magnetic field or radiation belts were discovered around the planet.

Section 32   Jupiter and Saturn

Observations of dark spots as they travel over the disk of Jupiter (Plate 10) serve to determine the planet's period of rotation on its axis. This period is not the same for the entire disk and amounts to 9^h51^m at the equator and 9^h56^m at the poles. This phenomenon of non-uniform (differential) rotation is also observed in the case of Saturn (Plate 11). It may, therefore, be concluded that the spots which we observe are not details of the actual surface of these planets but occur in their atmospheres. Just as Venus, Jupiter and Saturn are enveloped in a dense atmosphere which prevents us from observing the surface of these planets. Strong bands of methane CH_4, ammonia NH_3, and carbon dioxide CO_2 are observed in the spectrum of light from these planets, but hydrogen and helium are probably the principal constituents of the atmospheres.

Jupiter is a powerful source of radio emission. Observations of radiation with wavelengths of a few centimetres yield values of 140–200°K for the atmospheric temperature and this is in agreement with evaluations using infrared measurements. Thus, this radiation is certainly of a thermal origin. However, the intensity of the radiation in the decimetre wavelength region is so high that the corresponding temperature of the Jovian atmosphere would have to attain values of several thousand degrees Kelvin; this radiation has also been found to be polarized. Thus, a different mechanism of emission must be responsible for this radiation. The most convincing explanation is that it is emitted by fast electrons spiralling along lines of force in the magnetic field of Jupiter (so-called synchrotron radiation). This would mean that belts of radiation similar to the Van Allen belts surrounding the Earth exist around Jupiter.

Section 33 Interplanetary Matter

Mass spectrometers carried by space vehicles far beyond the Earth's magnetic field have recorded that a stream of ions with an intensity of 10^8 particles/cm$^2 \cdot$ sec flows away from the Sun. The velocity of these particles is about 500 km/sec but at times exceeds 1000 km/sec. This phenomenon, called the "solar wind," is due to turbulent processes in the solar atmosphere. They cause heating of the solar corona (Cf. Sec. 36) where the temperature reaches millions of degrees. When it is subjected to such violent heating, the corona is incapable of radiating the energy supplied it or transferring it to the interplanetary medium by thermal conduction. Consequently, it must expand out into space, carrying matter and the energy contained in it. For this reason there is no sharp boundary at which the solar corona ends. It even seems that the entire interplanetary space may be treated as the outer part of the corona in which the planets and their atmospheres are immersed. As a result, exchange of matter and a flow of heat can take place between the outer parts of the planetary atmospheres and the corona. The flow of energy directly from the solar corona to the upper layers of planetary atmospheres is probably one reason why the temperature increases with altitude in the terrestrial atmosphere at heights exceeding 85 km above sea level.

Violent explosions on the Sun are accompanied by the ejection of large clouds of ionized gas into space. These clouds move under the joint action of the solar gravitational field and the interplanetary magnetic field which stretches far into space. The passage of such a cloud close to the Earth causes perturbations in the terrestrial magnetosphere.

The existence of dust in interplanetary space is indicated by observations of the zodiacal light. A pale light stretching in a belt approximately along the ecliptic is visible against the background of the dark sky (especially just after dusk or just before dawn in the equatorial regions where the plane of the ecliptic is at a large angle to the plane of the horizon).

The surface brightness of various parts of this belt depends on the position of the Sun. The spectrum of zodiacal light is a reflection of the spectrum of sunlight, with the same distribution of Fraunhofer lines. This indicates that zodiacal light is due to solar radiation being scattered by grains of dust present in a narrow layer around the plane of the ecliptic.

Apart from minute grains of dust, there are solids of larger dimensions in interplanetary space. The largest are called planetoids. These are solid bodies travelling around the Sun in elliptical orbits, mainly between the orbits of Mars and Jupiter (only a small number of planetoids approaches the Sun at their perihelion to a distance less than that of the Earth). The diameters of the largest planetoids do not exceed several hundred kilometres (the largest is Ceres which is 770 km in diameter); most of the known planetoids have diameters of several or several tens of kilometres. It is difficult to speak of a lower limit on the size of planetoids. The smallest, probably coming into being continuously as the result of larger ones breaking up during collision with each other, reflect too little light to be observed. They may then be classified in the category of small bodies which we call meteors.

It frequently happens that the path of a meteor intersects the orbit of the Earth and the meteor enters the atmosphere. Such an event is commonly referred to as "a falling star". During its flight through the atmosphere, the meteor conveys its kinetic energy to air molecules which are thus excited to glow. At the same time, the meteor itself heats up. In most cases the meteor melts and vaporizes in the atmosphere. Only the largest reach the ground. Study of the chemical composition of meteorites (the name given to chunks of meteors which fall upon the ground) leads to their classification in three categories: stony, iron-stony, and iron meteorites. The first is made up mainly of silicates, while the latter consist primarily (about 95%) of iron and nickel. Iron-stony meteorites are an intermediate group in regard to chemical composition.

Comets comprise a separate group of bodies in interplanetary space. They consist of a nucleus (a swarm of particles, or one or several solid masses) and a gas and dust envelope which usually stretches into the cometary coma containing the nucleus and an extended cometary tail. The shape, size, and brightness of a comet vary considerably even during a single passage of the comet around the Sun. Cometary tails observed with the unaided eye stretch for several million kilometres, but there are even longer ones which attain lengths of hundreds of millions of kilometres. Notwithstanding their considerable size, comets have small masses— probably several orders of magnitude smaller than the masses of the planets since comets have not been found to cause perturbations in the motions of the other bodies in the solar system. The disintegration of comets, which is sometimes observed to occur, leads to the formation of meteor streams moving in orbits close to the original orbit of the comet. This is no doubt one of the sources of meteors in interplanetary space.

Chapter 4 Stellar Structure

The energy conditions on Earth and in its atmosphere are determined by the energy flux from the Sun. In later chapters we shall see that the energy radiated by the stars is decisive in regard to the conditions in interstellar matter. Indeed, stars prove to be the most productive suppliers of energy in most of the phenomena observed by astronomers. It is thus vitally important to be aware of the essence of the processes in which energy is produced in stars and then emitted into space as electromagnetic radiation.

Unfortunately, observation provides us with information only about the structure of the atmospheres or outer layers of stars. The inner parts, which are responsible for the production of energy, are shrouded in opaque atmospheres and thus cannot be observed directly. Instead, they can merely be studied theoretically. Presentation of a description of the inner layers of a star, one that is not contrary to present physical knowledge and which explains the facts observed in its atmosphere (its structure, the energy flux through it, etc.) can be treated as a solution to the problem of stellar structure.

The structure of the stellar atmosphere will be discussed in the first part of this chapter while the fundamentals of internal structure will be presented in later sections.

THE SOLAR ATMOSPHERE

The best known stellar atmosphere is that of the Sun. The Sun is the only star whose surface is visible as a disk. This makes it possible to study the structure of that surface, to learn the structure of the atmosphere, and to make a closer examination of the processes occurring in it. Furthermore, the Sun is an example of a typical stationary star (this is the term we shall use to denote a star whose brightness and internal structure do not vary with time; this does not mean, of course, that we exclude the possibility of slow evolutionary changes in such stars) and its atmosphere may be regarded as being typical, similar to the atmospheres of a vast multitude of stars in the Galaxy. For these reasons we shall confine ourselves in this chapter to discussing the solar atmosphere as an example of stellar atmospheres. It should be borne in mind, however, that the atmospheres of many stars differ substantially from that of the Sun. In most cases this is due to the different internal structure of these stars.

Section 34   The Structure of the Photosphere

The photosphere is the name given to the deepest layer of the solar atmosphere visible to the naked eye. This is the layer which accounts for almost all of the visible radiation arriving directly at the Earth. As a result of the opacity of the gas of which the Sun is composed, radiation emitted from the interior of the Sun is absorbed in overlying layers and is subsequently transmitted to layers further from the centre in emissions. Because of this process, the spectral distribution of the radiation changes with distance from the centre of the Sun since it is determined by the conditions obtaining in the layer from which this radiation was last emitted. This process continues until the radiation reaches the photosphere, where it is emitted directly into space. Thus the observed spectral distribution of the radiation of the Sun in the visible region is determined primarily by the conditions in the photosphere.

The so-called solar constant S is a measure of the total radiant energy emitted per unit time by the Sun. This unit is used for the energy of solar radiation incident perpendicularly upon 1 cm^2 of the Earth in one minute. Measurements of the solar constant (after allowing for losses in the Earth's atmosphere) give a value of

$$S = 1.95 \text{ cal} \cdot \text{cm}^{-2} \cdot \text{min}^{-1}. \tag{4-1}$$

If the distance between the Earth and the Sun is denoted by d, then

$$L = 4\pi d^2 S = 3.82 \times 10^{33} \text{ erg} \cdot \text{sec}^{-1} \tag{4-2}$$

is the energy which flows per second through the surface of a sphere of radius equal to that of the Earth's orbit. This energy must be equal to that which leaves the surface of the Sun per second. Hence, each square centimetre of solar surface emits energy at the rate of

$$I = \frac{L}{4\pi R_\odot^2} = 6.28 \times 10^{10} \text{ erg} \cdot \text{cm}^{-2} \cdot \text{sec}^{-1}, \tag{4-3}$$

where $R_\odot = 6.96 \times 10^{10}$ cm is the solar radius. The amount of energy emitted by the surface of some body per cm^2 per sec depends on the temperature of that body. If as a first approximation we assume that the spectral distribution of the sunlight is given by Planck's radiation formula [Cf. Chap. 3, Eq. (3-93)], then (as is readily seen upon integrating both sides of Planck's formula with respect to λ from 0 to ∞) we have

$$I = \sigma T^4, \tag{4-4}$$

where $\sigma = 5.67 \times 10^{-5}$ erg $\cdot$ cm$^{-2} \cdot$ sec$^{-1} \cdot$ deg^{-4} is the Stefan–Boltzmann constant. Equation (4-4) is the Stefan–Boltzmann law.

The temperature found from the Stefan–Boltzmann law is called the effective temperature. Thus, the effective temperature T_e of the photo-sphere is

$$T_e = \sqrt[4]{\frac{I}{\sigma}} = \sqrt[4]{\frac{6.28 \times 10^{10}}{5.67 \times 10^5}} \times 1°K = 5770°K. \qquad (4\text{-}5)$$

Of course the temperature of the photosphere varies with altitude. For this reason the temperature of the individual layers of the photosphere differs from the effective temperature we have found. However, the effective temperature may be treated as a sort of mean temperature of the photosphere or as the temperature of that photosphere layer which emits the largest fraction of radiation arriving directly at the Earth.

At various places on the Sun's disk the position of the layer whose visible radiation is emitted directly towards the Earth is not the same. As we look at the solar limb, the light rays traverse the photosphere layers obliquely and in consequence radiation from layers closer to the upper surface of the photosphere reach the observer than during observation of the middle of the Sun's disk (Cf. Fig. 4-1). Therefore the radiation

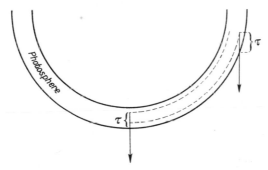

Figure 4-1. The position of layers from which radiation emitted by the centre and edge of the solar disk arrives.

arriving from various points on the Sun's disk comes from layers at various depths in the photosphere: as we observe areas which are more and more remote from the middle of the disk, we receive light emitted from higher and higher layers. Figure 4-2 gives the distribution of the surface brightness along the diameter of the solar disk for radiation of wavelengths 3300 Å, 6689 Å, 12,475 Å, 22,189 Å. Darkening towards the solar limb can be seen in the plot. This phenomenon, which also occurs in the atmospheres of other celestial bodies, is called limb darkening. Since the intensity of the radiation from higher layers of the photosphere (radiation from the limb) is less than that of radiation from lower-lying layers (centre of the disk), it may be said in accordance with the Stefan–Boltzmann law that the temperature of the deeper layers of the photosphere is higher than

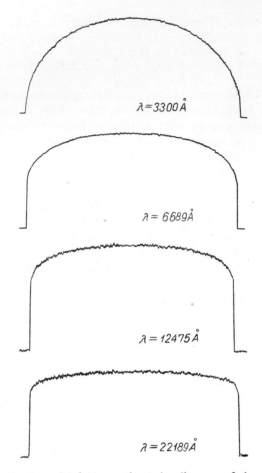

Figure 4-2. Distribution of brightness along the diameter of the solar disk for various wavelength [After Peyturaux, *Ann. d'Astrophys.* **18,** 34 (1955)].

that of the outer layers, i.e. that the temperature in the photosphere decreases towards the top. The temperature of the uppermost surface of the photosphere is of the order of 4500°K.

The chemical composition of the solar atmosphere can be determined by observation of the solar spectrum (Plate 12). In order to elucidate this, we must consider how the observed spectral distribution of the radiation is produced in the solar atmosphere.

As we shall see later, hydrogen and helium are the principal components of the solar atmosphere. At 4500° to 6000°K neither of these elements is ionized, and the helium atoms even remain unexcited. However, the heavier elements whose ionization potentials are much lower do undergo ionization. Some of the free electrons combine with the neutral hydrogen atoms to form negative hydrogen ions H^-. Under the influence of radiation there may be disintegration of the negative hydrogen ion with the simultaneous absorption of a photon whose energy is used in part to overcome the forces binding the electron with the hydrogen atom and in part to impart kinetic energy to the electron so freed and to the neutral hydrogen atom. During close approaches the electrons exchange kinetic energy with each other and with the ions. As a result a certain energy distribution of free electrons is established. Their mean energy determines the temperature of the medium. If a free electron is bound once again with a neutral hydrogen atom, a photon is emitted. The energy of the emitted photon, however, is in general different from the energy of the photon previously absorbed when that electron was being released from a negative hydrogen ion, since the energy distribution of photons emitted during the production of negative hydrogen ions is determined by the energy distribution of free electrons in the medium, and hence is determined by the photosphere temperature. A continuous spectrum thus is produced in the photosphere.

Generally speaking, a continuous spectrum of solar radiation will be produced as a result of all sorts of recombination processes in the medium. Account must thus be taken here of recombination with metal ions as well as with ionized hydrogen atoms, a number of which might be produced in the medium owing to ionization of neutral hydrogen atoms previously excited to a higher-lying state (the energy required to ionize an excited atom is less than the ionization energy of an atom in the ground state). However, the influence of both these processes on the formation of a continuous spectrum of solar radiation is negligible.

Neutral hydrogen atoms, and metal ions are subjected to excitation upon absorbing photons of particular energies. An electron then jumps from a lower energy level to a higher one. The energy of the absorbed photon is exactly equal to the potential difference between the two energy levels. It is true that the reverse process corresponds to this: during the jump of electrons from higher energy levels to lower ones, excited atoms emit photons of energies characteristic for the given atom and excited state, but these photons are radiated in an arbitrary direction, generally not the same as the original one. This means that photons of energies which can be absorbed during excitation of atoms and ions of the medium are scattered repeatedly and in effect they wander in the photosphere for a much longer time than do photons of other energies. Many of them may be absorbed by negative hydrogen ions and their energy is then passed on to electrons freed from the H^- ions and subsequently emitted in a continuous spectrum as described earlier. In this way, some of the photons of energy equal to the excitation energy of the atoms and ions are eliminared from the continuous spectrum and absorption lines are produced in the photosphere.

The intensity of a spectral line depends on, among other things, the density of atoms (or ions) capable of absorbing photons of an energy corresponding to that line, i.e. on the density of atoms (or ions) of a particular element in a particular excited state. Measurement of the intensity of Fraunhofer lines observed in the solar spectrum may thus serve to determine these densities. On the other hand, knowing the conditions in the photosphere (temperature, pressure), we can find the relative number of atoms excited to successive energy states as compared to the aggregate number of atoms of the given element. Thus, in consequence the chemical composition of the solar photosphere can be determined on the basis of observation of spectral lines. The results are listed in Table 4-1.

TABLE 4-1

Chemical Composition of the Solar Atmosphere

Constituent	Percentage Abundance by Mass
Hydrogen H	72.7
Helium He	26.2
Oxygen O	0.69
Carbon C	0.31
Nitrogen N	0.06

In addition to the elements mentioned above, most of those which occur on Earth have been detected in the solar atmosphere; these include magnesium, silicon, sulphur, iron, calcium, nickel, sodium, and aluminium. The solar atmosphere has also been found to contain some molecules (above all, molecules of unsaturated compounds), such as CN, OH, CH, NH.

The thickness of the photosphere is given by the magnitude of the transmission coefficient. As we go deeper into the photosphere an ever smaller fraction of the light emitted there leaves the Sun and the rest is re-absorbed in the overlying layers. Almost all of the visible radiation arrives from a layer some 300 km thick and it is this which may be regarded as the thickness of the photosphere. Though its optical thickness is great, the density of the photosphere is less than that in the Earth's atmosphere at sea level by a factor of several thousand to several million; namely, at the upper surface of the photosphere it is less than 10^{-9} g·cm^{-3} whereas at the base of the photosphere it increases to several times 10^{-7} g·cm^{-3}.

The photosphere surface is not homogeneous. Distinct granulation can be seen on the solar disk. Against the background of the somewhat darker disk are small areas, called granulae, of increased brightness (Plate 13). The observed granula diameters vary from 200 km to 2000 km. Granulae, which appear over the entire surface of the Sun, are short-lived and each disappears within several minutes. Measurement of the velocity of granulae leads to the conclusion that they move with respect to the surrounding medium in a direction perpendicular to the photosphere surface with mean velocities of the order of 1/3 km per sec. The temperature of granulae, as indicated by comparison of surface brightnesses, is about 100 degrees higher than the temperature of the remaining regions of the photosphere.

The presence of granulae testifies to the fact that the photosphere has turbulent motion which causes gas from the hotter layers underlying the photosphere to be ejected upwards into the photosphere. In this way heat is transferred along with matter into the outer layers of the photosphere. This mechanism of energy transport by convection in the photosphere however is much less effective than the energy transport by radiation as described above. The sources of turbulent motions in the photosphere, of which granulae are a manifestation, are associated with the structure of the layers underlying the photosphere and will therefore be discussed in Sec. 41.

Section 35   The Structure of the Chromosphere

During total eclipses, when the Moon covers the Sun's disk, the outer layers of the solar atmosphere—the chromosphere and the corona—can be observed. The lower-lying layer, the chromosphere, is then visible as a red ring around the dark solar disk. The spectrum of the chromosphere (Plate 14) is seen to have emission lines against the background of a weak continuous spectrum. The arrangement of these lines, especially in radiation from the lower parts of the chromosphere, is reminiscent of the Fraunhofer lines. The difference consists primarily in the occurrence of lines of atoms excited to higher energy levels than in the photosphere; for instance, we observe helium lines which do not appear in the radiation of the photosphere. These differences increase with height in the chromosphere.

The presence of atoms excited to high energy levels is evidence of the high temperature in the chromosphere, higher than in the photosphere. Thus, the temperature of the solar atmosphere at the surface dividing the photosphere and chromosphere attains a minimum of the order of 4500°K and increases in both directions, downwards as we go deeper into the photosphere, and upwards in the chromosphere.

Estimates of the chromosphere temperature on the basis of the lines of various elements lead to differing results. For instance, strong hydrogen and helium lines are seen to appear at one height. And yet, the energy required to excite a helium atom is about $1\frac{1}{2}$ times the ionization energy of the hydrogen atom. At the temperature at which helium can glow (it must be excited to do this), hydrogen will have been almost completely ionized and thus spectral lines of this element should not appear; conversely, at lower temperatures at which hydrogen is not ionized and produces spectral lines, helium atoms remain unexcited. It is a similar story in the case of the lines of other elements. Thus it follows that the thermal conditions in the chromosphere cannot be described by means of a single parameter characterizing the temperature. This points to the absence of thermodynamic equilibrium in the chromosphere. A model treating the chromosphere as a medium consisting of two constituents, hot and cold, may be used as the simplest model for describing the chromosphere. In using such a model, we must give two sets of values of temperature, density, etc., one for the colder regions and one for the hotter regions, for each height in the chromosphere.

Splashes of material, so-called spicules, at times reaching an altitude of 10,000 km above the base of the chromosphere, are ejected from the lower reaches of the chromosphere. These spicules make the chromosphere look like burning prairie (Fig. 4-3). Material from the lower layers

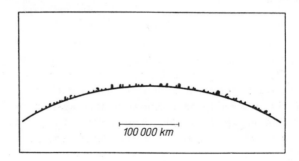

Figure 4-3. Chromospheric spicules.

of the chromosphere is carried upwards in these spicules and thus, because a temperature gradient exists in the upper layers of the chromosphere, regions which differ substantially from each other in temperature are formed.

Measurements of the radio-frequency radiation from the Sun may also be employed to determine the chromosphere temperature. It has been stated earlier (Cf. Sec. 26) that a medium of high electron density is opaque to radio radiation of wavelengths longer than a limiting value. The value of this limiting wavelength decreases with the increase in the electron density of the medium. Thus, the longer the wavelength of the radio radiation received, the higher (more rarefied) the layer of the solar atmosphere that this radiation comes from. Knowing the intensity of the radio radiation for various wavelengths, we can estimate the temperature of the chromosphere at various altitudes. Measurements of radiation of wavelengths of the order of 1 cm originating in the central layers of the chromosphere lead to temperatures not exceeding 10,000°K. The temperatures estimated on the basis of radiation of longer wavelengths are higher; for waves of several centimetres the temperatures are about 20,000°K, while metre waves coming from the outer parts of the chromosphere and the deep layers of the corona indicate that a temperature of the order of 100,000 to 1,000,000°K exists there.

Additional information about the chromosphere is obtained by extra-atmospheric investigations of solar radiation in the far ultraviolet (Fig. 4-4). Although the optical thickness of layers overlying the photosphere

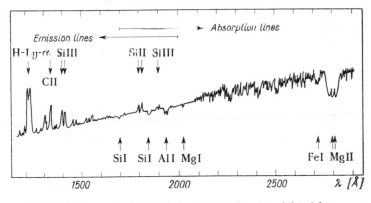

Figure 4-4. The spectrum of solar radiation in the far ultraviolet (plot of intensity vs. wavelength).

for visible radiation is small (for $\lambda = 5000$ Å, $\tau = 0.02$), the coefficient of absorption nevertheless increases rapidly with a decrease in wavelength. For this reason, radiation of wavelengths shorter than 1700 Å comes entirely from the chromosphere. The most conspicuous feature of the solar spectrum in this wave range is the occurrence of the emission lines of hydrogen, and of the highly ionized atoms of such elements as oxygen, iron, silicon, calcium, carbon, and others, including ionized and neutral helium.

The presence of emission lines in the ultraviolet region of the solar spectrum is a consequence of the rise in temperature with the altitude in the chromosphere. Since the coefficient of absorption for light of wavelengths corresponding to the spectral lines is larger than for other wavelengths, the radiation in the lines comes from higher, and hence hotter, layers of the chromosphere than does radiation in the continuous spectrum. Here, the situation is the reverse of that for radiation from the photosphere, where lines were produced in the cooler layers.

The rise in the temperature from about 4500°K at the base of the chromosphere to several hundred thousand degrees at an altitude of 10,000 km cannot be due to the flow of radiant energy from the photosphere since this energy flow lacks photons of sufficient energy to ionize hydrogen and helium. On the other hand, energy cannot flow into the chromosphere by conduction from the photosphere to overlying layers since heat can flow only from a hotter to a colder medium. Thus, the heat flow from the photosphere, directly or via radiation, cannot be what causes the chromosphere to heat up. This compels us to seek other sources of heat for the chromosphere. The only forms of energy which may be converted into thermal energy of the chromosphere are: the kinetic energy of gas and the energy of the solar magnetic field. Under certain circumstances, the gaseous motions occurring in the chromosphere may be dissipated as heat. We have already spoken of turbulence in the photosphere; granulae are manifestations of it. Such motions may propagate upwards to the chromosphere, causing sound waves to propagate in the upper layers of the solar atmosphere. As the density of the medium diminishes, the amplitude of these waves increases and the waves become shock waves. The propagation of shock waves is accompanied by strong dissipation of kinetic energy owing to the collision of atoms moving in the wavefront with atoms of the medium through which the waves are sweeping. This causes the chromosphere to heat up. The motion of ionized gas in the chromosphere is strongly linked with the magnetic field occurring in the chromosphere. As a result of interactions between the moving material and the magnetic field, an exchange of kinetic and magnetic energy may occur. At the same time, the energy of the magnetic field may be dissipated as heat when electrons and ions accelerated by the magnetic field collide with each other and with neutral atoms.

The thermal conditions in the chromosphere depend not only on processes which result in energy being supplied to the medium but also on processes leading to irradiation of energy. The efficiency of the latter, however, is small in view of the low density of the chromosphere. Thus, the energy flux carried in shock waves, required to heat the chromosphere to the temperatures observed in it, need not be large. In actual fact, it is several orders of magnitude smaller than the flux of radiant energy from the photosphere through the chromosphere which displays almost complete transparency to this radiation.

Section 36   The Solar Corona

The outermost part of the solar atmosphere is called the corona. It stretches far above the chromosphere, reaching all the way to the Earth's orbit. The inner part of the corona can be seen during solar eclipse as a solar aureole around the eclipsing disk of the Moon. The shape and size of the corona depend on the phase of the solar cycle (Cf. Sec. 37). At activity maximum it is more extensive and spherical, while apart from the maximum it becomes flattened along the equator (Plate 15).

The heating of the lower corona is due to the same processes which determine the temperature in the chromosphere, the dissipation of shock waves. Owing to the low density of the gas, of the order of 10^{-15} g $\cdot$ cm^{-3} at the base of the corona, energy is radiated at a slow rate; the energy efflux due to thermal conduction is also not highly effective. The result is that the corona temperature reaches 1,000,000–2,000,000°K, and energy transport out of the Sun must take place by convection—the outflow of hot gas from the corona into interplanetary space ("solar wind"; Cf. Sec. 33).

This means that the matter comprising the corona is continuously being carried away from the Sun in the "solar wind" and at the same time the corona is continuously renewed with gas flowing in from the chromosphere (the period which matter takes to flow through the corona amounts to several weeks). This is why the solar corona has no outer limit. With distance from the Sun, the density of the corona (solar wind) gradually decreases, to fall off to a value of the order of several tens of ions per cm^3 at a distance of 1 AU.

Section 37   Solar Activity

The structure of the solar atmosphere, as described in the preceding section, characterizes what is known as "the quiet Sun". However, a number of phenomena hitherto not discussed occur in the surface layers of the Sun. These phenomena as a whole, which consist of such phenomena as spots and faculae in the photosphere, flares and prominences in the chromosphere, as well as the shape and size of the corona, are called solar activity. The intensity of these phenomena is subject to periodic fluctuations, reaching a maximum at intervals of more or less 11 years. For this reason, we speak of the 11-year cycle of solar activity.

Sunspots (Plate 16) are those manifestations of solar activity which have been known and investigated the longest. These are regions of the order of 10,000 km in size (some are smaller), darker and thus cooler (by some 1000°K) than the surrounding photosphere. In general, sunspots appear in groups. Most frequently, groups of spots disappear two days or so after they first appear. However, the lifetime of some, especially larger ones, runs to several tens of days, or even a hundred days. The number of spots, their position on the solar disk, and their lifetime are related to the phase of solar activity. The moment when the largest number of spots appear on the solar disk is treated as the maximum solar activity. From that moment on, the number of spots gradually decreases, falling off by an average factor of twenty during a minimum. Spots occur only near the solar equator*, in a belt of width $\pm 35°$ on either side of it.

Sunspots are accompanied by faculae, regions which are somewhat brighter than the surrounding photosphere. Faculae are best observable far from the centre of the solar disk; they seem to be fewer in number near the centre. This indicates that faculae are phenomena which occur in the upper layers of the photosphere and therefore, when our sight reaches out to the deeper layers (hotter layers), the faculae disappear against the background of those layers.

Solar spots and faculae form active regions on the Sun's disk. Strong magnetic fields are detected in these regions and in spots the field intensities go as high as 2000 to 3000 oersteds. The occurrence of a magnetic field is the first sign that an active region is being created. This field also persists for some time after a spot has disappeared in a given region. The strong magnetic field affects the motion of the matter in which it occurs. In particular, rapid small scale turbulent motions are damped and the pressure distribution in the photosphere also changes since magnetic pressure appears in these regions in addition to the gas pressure. This causes imbalance in the photosphere, thus leading to deviations of the temperature and brightness of the active regions and to the production of sunspots and faculae in the photosphere.

The magnetic field from the active regions of the photosphere penetrates into the uppermost layers of the solar atmosphere. In these layers (of much lower density) this field may induce motions of material and energy of these motions may then be dissipated as heat.

In fact, above the active regions we observe so-called chromospheric flares which are evident on spectroheliograms in lines originating in the chromosphere (Plate 17). These are very short-lived formations: after reaching maximum brightness within a few minutes they disappear in a short time (not exceeding 2 hours for the largest flares). Most frequently, flares appear over groups of sunspots possessing a complex structure of magnetic field, especially in periods when the field experiences rapid changes.

The existence of prominences is also undoubtedly associated with the presence of magnetic fields in the solar atmosphere. These are bright objects ejected to an altitude of tens of thousands of kilometres above

* The solar equatorial plane is a plane passing through the centre of the Sun and perpendicular to the rotational axis of the Sun. The inclination of the solar equator to the ecliptic is 7° 15′.

the surface of the chromosphere. Their length not infrequently runs to 200,000 km. A photograph of a prominence is shown in Plate 18. The number of prominences depends on the phase of the solar cycle, but the fluctuations in this number are smaller than those in the number of sunspots.

The phase of the solar cycle bears no effect on the magnitude of the total energy flux from the Sun. Measurements of the solar constant do not indicate the existence of observed fluctuations of this constant during a cycle. Some changes may only occur for radiation in the far ultraviolet and in the radio frequency band; however, the energy of this radiation emitted in the chromosphere and the corona is several orders of magnitude smaller than in the visible region and thus these fluctuations do not affect the constancy of the total flux of solar energy. The fact that the energy emitted by the Sun is constant indicates that phenomena associated with the solar cycle do not affect the rate of energy production, and hence do not reach those central parts of the Sun in which that production takes place.

The magnetic field plays a vital role in the formation of active regions. Thus, the causes of solar activity should be sought among phenomena which can alter the topography of that field inside the Sun and bring it towards the surface. An important role is certainly played here by the non-uniform rotation of the Sun, among other things, as testified to by the formation of active regions about the solar equator.

THE INTERNAL STRUCTURE OF STARS

The purpose of the following sections is to present the fundamentals of the internal structure of stars. Observational data in most cases concern parameters which specify the star as a whole, such as the mass $\mathfrak{M}$, the radius R, and the amount of energy L emitted by the star per unit time. These observational data must suffice for determining the processes taking place inside the stars. The structure of the stellar interiors will be considered here for the simplest case of a single, non-rotating star of constant brightness. It will also be assumed that the star does not have a magnetic field.

Section 38   Spherical Symmetry and the Hydrostatic Equilibrium of Stars

In order to describe the structure of a star, it is necessary—among other things—to give for every point in its interior the value of the density ϱ, pressure p, temperature T, and possibly other parameters as well. In general, ϱ, p, and T are functions of the time t and three spatial coordinates x, y, z in some arbitrary rectangular system

$$\varrho = \varrho(x, y, z, t), \tag{4-6}$$

$$p = p(x, y, z, t), \tag{4-7}$$

$$T = T(x, y, z, t). \tag{4-8}$$

The restriction of our considerations to single, non-rotating stars, devoid of any internal magnetic field, means assuming the absence of factors which could cause the star to lose its spherical symmetry. Otherwise, when a star rotates, for instance, a centrifugal force acts on the stellar matter. This force causes a surface of equal density (ϱ = const) to be flattened along the axis of rotation. In the case of multiple systems, surfaces of equal density may be deformed by the action of gravitational forces from other stars in the system. A strong internal magnetic field could also destroy the spherical symmetry of a star. However, if we confine ourselves to stars possessing spherical symmetry, all the parameters describing the state of the matter will be functions only of the distance r from the centre of the star and the time t:

$$\varrho = \varrho(r, t), \tag{4-9}$$

$$p = p(r, t), \tag{4-10}$$

$$T = T(r, t). \tag{4-11}$$

Let $S(r)$ denote a sphere of radius r which is concentric with the star (Fig. 4-5). Let $M(r, t)$ be the mass contained inside the sphere $S(r)$. This mass is expressed by the volume integral

$$M(r, t) = \int_{S(r)} \varrho(r, t) dV. \tag{4-12}$$

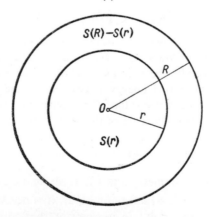

Figure 4-5. Cross section of a star and the sphere $S(r)$.

Since the star is spherically symmetric, the differential dV can be expressed in terms of the differential dr

$$dV = 4\pi r^2 dr. \tag{4-13}$$

Therefore

$$M(r, t) = \int_0^r \varrho(r, t) 4\pi r^2 dr. \tag{4-14}$$

Differentiating Eq. (4-14), we can rewrite the relation between $M(r, t)$ and $\varrho(r, t)$ as a differential equation

$$\frac{\partial M(r, t)}{\partial r} = 4\pi \varrho(r, t) r^2. \tag{4-15}$$

Let us now use the assumption that the star under consideration is stationary, i.e., its brightness and radius are constant. From this we conclude that the structure of the interior of the star does not vary with time (ϱ, p, T, M are functions only of r). The necessary condition for such a state is that the sum of forces acting on the matter at any point in the star vanish, i.e. hydrostatic equilibrium exist in the star. Inasmuch as we have excluded magnetic, centrifugal, and external forces acting on the star, our problem reduces to one of considering the dependence of the pressure on internal gravitational forces.

Let $g(r)$ denote the gravitational acceleration at the surface of a sphere $S(r)$. In view of the spherical symmetry of the star, this acceleration is directed towards the centre of the star (it has only a component parallel to the radius vector of the given point). Thus, we can use Eq. (3-79') to write

$$\frac{dp(r)}{dr} = -g(r)\varrho(r). \tag{4-16}$$

To calculate the gravitational acceleration $g(r)$ at the surface of the sphere $S(r)$, let us divide the star into two parts: the first part will constitute the sphere $S(r)$, while the other part will comprise the rest of the star—a spherical layer $S(R)-S(r)$ (Cf. Fig. 4-5). The acceleration due to gravity at the surface of the sphere is equal to the acceleration evoked by the attraction from a material point (particle) equal in mass to the sphere and placed at the centre of symmetry. Thus, the gravitational acceleration due to the matter contained inside the sphere $S(r)$ is equal to $GM(r)/r^2$. On the other hand, the gravitational accelerations due to various parts of the layer $S(R)-S(r)$ cancel at all points of the sphere $S(r)$. Therefore, the layer $S(R)-S(r)$ does not make any contribution to the acceleration at points lying on the surface of sphere $S(r)$ and the total acceleration at those points is

$$g(r) = \frac{GM(r)}{r^2}. \tag{4-17}$$

Thus, the equation describing the hydrostatic equilibrium in the star assumes the form

$$\frac{dp(r)}{dr} = -\frac{GM(r)}{r^2}\varrho(r). \tag{4-18}$$

We shall rewrite Eq. (4-15) here as

$$\frac{dM(r)}{dr} = 4\pi\varrho(r)r^2 \tag{4-19}$$

since in a stationary star both M and ϱ do not depend on time. Equations (4-15) and (4-19) are the first two equations for the internal structure of the star.

Section 39   The Equation of State

The temperature in the interior of a star cannot be lower than the temperature of the photosphere. As we shall soon see, it is indeed much higher. Under these conditions matter can occur only in the form of gas.

Considering stars similar in structure to the Sun, we can treat the stellar gas as an ideal gas. However, in many stars (e.g. white dwarfs—Cf. Sec. 54) the density of the matter is so high (in excess of 10^3 g·cm^{-3}) that the gas loses the properties of an ideal gas and becomes a degenerate gas. This is due to the fact that when the separation between molecules is small, we must take account of the quantum-mechanical principle known as the Pauli exclusion principle which states that no more than one particle can be in a given quantum state. By quantum state we mean the complete set of parameters specifying the position and motion of a particle. When the density in the medium is high, the Pauli principle introduces a restriction on the motion of electrons in the medium, thus making the ideal gas law inapplicable. A characteristic feature of degenerate gas is that small variations in density cause much greater changes of pressure than in the case of an ideal gas and that the gas pressure depends only slightly on the temperature. Such a gas is much less compressible than is an ideal gas. Thus, a different equation of state relating the pressure to the density must be used for degenerate gases.

In the case of stars with even higher densities (of the order of 10^{12} g·cm^{-3} and higher), reconstruction of the particles of the stellar matter ensues. At such high densities, electrons combine with protons into neutrons and we then have a gas composed of neutrons, and not of atoms as is the case in stars of densities comparable to that of the Sun. Such stars are called neutron stars (Cf. Sec. 54). Owing to their high density, when considering the internal structure of neutron stars we must replace Eq. (4-18) by an equation of hydrostatic equilibrium which takes relativistic effects into account. The equation of state also takes on a form different from that for the ideal gas.

For the time being, however, let us confine ourselves to consideration of stars in which the gas is nondegenerate. We can then employ the equation of state for ideal gases

$$p(r) = \frac{\mathscr{R}}{\mu} \varrho(r) T(r), \tag{4-20}$$

where $\mathscr{R} = 8.314 \times 10^7$ cm$^2 \cdot$ sec$^{-2} \cdot$ deg^{-1} is a gas constant, and μ is the mean molecular mass expressed in units of mass of the hydrogen atom.

The mean molecular mass μ depends, of course, on the chemical composition of the medium. As we saw when discussing the atmosphere of the Sun, hydrogen and helium are the most abundant elements in stars. Let X denote the ratio of the mass of hydrogen to the total mass contained in a unit volume, Y the same ratio for helium, and Z for other, heavier elements. Of course

$$X + Y + Z = 1. \tag{4-21}$$

Let us now find the mean molecular mass as a function of X, Y, Z. Since inside stars (with the exception of their atmosphere and sub-photospheric layers) all atoms are completely ionized (only the ions of heavy elements may retain electrons in inner orbits), two particles (one electron and one proton) come into being from each hydrogen atom, three particles (2 electrons and an alpha particle) from each helium atom, while about $\frac{1}{2}A$ particles are formed from each atom of heavier elements of atomic mass A. (The number of electrons for these heavier elements is approximately half the atomic mass; e.g. the atomic mass of carbon is 12.0, and the number of electrons in the atom is 6, for nitrogen these figures are, respectively, 14.0 and 7, for oxygen 16.0 and 8, etc.). Now let us calculate the number of particles in each cm^3. The mass of hydrogen contained in 1 cm^3 of the star is equal to $X\varrho$. If by m_H we denote the mass of the hydrogen atom, there will be $X\varrho/m_\mathrm{H}$ hydrogen atoms in this volume. The ionization of each atom of hydrogen will yield 2 particles and hence each cm^3 of the medium contains $2X\varrho/m_\mathrm{H}$ particles formed by the ionization of hydrogen atoms. In similar manner we can calculate that each cm^3 will have $\frac{3}{4}Y\varrho/m_\mathrm{H}$ particles originating from the ionization of helium and $\frac{1}{2}Z\varrho/m_\mathrm{H}$ particles from the ionization of heavy elements. Thus, the number of particles in each cm^3 is

$$N = 2X\frac{\varrho}{m_\mathrm{H}} + \frac{3}{4}Y\frac{\varrho}{m_\mathrm{H}} + \frac{1}{2}Z\frac{\varrho}{m_\mathrm{H}} = (2X + \frac{3}{4}Y + \frac{1}{2}Z)\frac{\varrho}{m_\mathrm{H}}. \tag{4-22}$$

The mean molecular mass in grams is equal to the mass contained in 1 cm^3 divided by the number of particles contained in that volume: ϱ/N. Thus, the molecular mass, expressed in terms of the atomic mass of hydrogen, is

$$\mu = \frac{\varrho}{Nm_\mathrm{H}} = (2X + \frac{3}{4}Y + \frac{1}{2}Z)^{-1}. \tag{4-23}$$

It is possible for X, Y, Z, and hence μ to be constant throughout the entire star. The star is then said to have a uniform chemical composition. Such a chemical composition can exist in general only in young stars since, as evolution proceeds, changes in the chemical composition can be expected to occur in the core of the star and μ then becomes a function of the distance r from the centre of the star.

The equation of state (4-20) takes account of pressure due only to the gas. In actual fact, the total pressure consists of the gas pressure and the radiation pressure. A term to describe the radiation pressure should, therefore, be added to Eq. (4-20). We shall not do this here since in the case of the Sun the radiation pressure does not exceed 3 per cent of the total pressure. It is necessary to take this term into account, however, when considering hotter, more massive stars. What has been said above by no means signifies that the existence of radiation pressure does not affect the structure of a star (even one like the Sun). We shall return to this topic in Sec. 41, when discussing the flow of radiation through a star.

Equations (4-18), (4-19), and (4-20) now provide a sufficient basis for evaluating some parameters which specify the conditions inside a star. Among other things, the mean temperature in the interior of a star can be evaluated from them.

The mean temperature $\overline{T}$ of some body of mass $\mathfrak{M}$, which consists of n parts such that the i-th part has a mass of m_i and a temperature of T_i, can be taken to be the expression

$$\overline{T} = \frac{\sum\limits_{i=1}^{n} T_i m_i}{\mathfrak{M}}. \tag{4-24}$$

If the number n of parts is increased infinitely so that in the process of division the mass of the largest part tends towards zero, the value obtained for the mean temperature will be

$$\overline{T} = \frac{1}{\mathfrak{M}} \int\limits_{0}^{\mathfrak{M}} T dM. \tag{4-25}$$

In relation to a star: $\mathfrak{M}$ denotes its mass, T the temperature at the surface of the sphere $S(r)$, dM the differential of mass contained in the sphere $S(r)$ [the mass contained in an infinitesimally thin layer $S(r+dr)-S(r)$ of the star].

When into the expression

$$\overline{T} = \frac{1}{\mathfrak{M}} \int\limits_{0}^{\mathfrak{M}} T(r) dM(r) \tag{4-26}$$

We substitute the temperature found from the equation of state (4-20)

$$T(r) = \frac{\mu p(r)}{\mathscr{R}\varrho(r)} \tag{4-27}$$

and the differential of mass

$$dM(r) = 4\pi\varrho(r)r^2 dr \tag{4-28}$$

calculated from Eq. (4-19), we have

$$\bar{T} = 4\pi \frac{1}{\mathfrak{M}} \frac{\mu}{\mathscr{R}} \int_0^R p(r)r^2 dr. \tag{4-29}$$

The integral in Eq. (4-29) is calculated piecewise

$$\int_0^R p(r)r^2 dr = [\tfrac{1}{3}p(r)r^3]_{r=0}^{r=R} - \frac{1}{3}\int_0^R r^3 \frac{dp(r)}{dr} dr. \tag{4-30}$$

The expression $[\tfrac{1}{3}p(r)r^3]_{r=0}^{r=R} = 0$, since at the surface of the star (for $r = R$) the pressure $p(r)$ vanishes, while at the centre $r^3 = 0$. Therefore

$$\bar{T} = -\frac{4\pi}{3} \frac{1}{\mathfrak{M}} \frac{\mu}{\mathscr{R}} \int_0^R r^3 \frac{dp(r)}{dr} dr. \tag{4-31}$$

If into Eq. (4-31) we insert $dp(r)/dr$ from the equation of hydrostatic equilibrium (4-18) and

$$dr = (4\pi\varrho(r)r^2)^{-1}dM(r) \tag{4-32}$$

from Eq. (4-19), we obtain

$$\bar{T} = \tfrac{1}{3} \frac{1}{\mathfrak{M}} \frac{\mu}{\mathscr{R}} G \int_0^{\mathfrak{M}} \frac{M(r)dM(r)}{r} = \tfrac{1}{6} \frac{1}{\mathfrak{M}} \frac{\mu}{\mathscr{R}} G \int_0^{\mathfrak{M}} \frac{d[M(r)]^2}{r}. \tag{4-33}$$

Without more precise information about the internal structure of the star [e.g. knowledge of the shape of the function $M(r)$] we cannot calculate the last integral. In any event, however, the value of this integral is underestimated if we replace r with the radius R of the star. We can then write

$$\bar{T} > \tfrac{1}{6} \frac{1}{\mathfrak{M}} \frac{\mu}{\mathscr{R}} \frac{G}{R} \int_0^{\mathfrak{M}} d[M(r)]^2 = \tfrac{1}{6} \frac{1}{\mathfrak{M}} \frac{\mu}{\mathscr{R}} \frac{G\mathfrak{M}^2}{R} = \tfrac{1}{6} \frac{\mu}{\mathscr{R}} \frac{G\mathfrak{M}}{R}. \tag{4-34}$$

If the values of the constants appearing here are inserted and if the mass and radius of the star are expressed in units of mass and radius of the Sun, inequality (4-34) can be rewritten as

$$\bar{T} > 3.8\times10^6 \mu \frac{\mathfrak{M}}{\mathfrak{M}_\odot} \frac{R_\odot}{R} \ (°K). \tag{4-35}$$

Since $\mu > \frac{1}{2}$ (why?), the mean temperature of the solar interior must exceed 1,900,000 degrees. However, since the temperature of the outer layers of stars is much lower than this value the temperature of the Sun's core must be substantially higher than the value obtained here for the mean temperature.

Section 40   Energy Production in Stars

At temperatures of several million degrees or higher thermonuclear reactions may occur in stars whereby nuclei of lighter elements combine into nuclei of heavier atoms. In order for these reactions to proceed, the reacting nuclei must approach each other sufficiently for the nuclear binding forces to come into play. We know, however, that two nuclei possessing Z_1 and Z_2 protons will repel each other with a force F determined by Coulomb's law

$$F = \frac{Z_1 Z_2 e^2}{d^2}, \tag{4-36}$$

where $e = 4.80 \times 10^{-10} \cdot \mathrm{g}^{\frac{1}{2}} \cdot \mathrm{cm}^{\frac{3}{2}} \cdot \mathrm{sec}^{-1}$ is the electric charge of the electron, and d is the separation of the nuclei. For the nuclei to collide, the energy E required to overcome the repulsive forces must be large enough, i.e.

$$E \geqslant E_0 = \frac{Z_1 Z_2 e^2}{d_0}, \tag{4-37}$$

where d_0 may be treated as the radius of the nucleus. This means that if the nuclear reactions are to occur, the velocities of the chaotic motions of the nuclei (hence, the temperature of the gas) must be high. Quantum mechanical considerations, it is true, do lead to the conclusion that even at lower temperatures (when the energy of the relative motion of the interacting nuclei is less than E_0) there is a nonzero probability of a nuclear reaction occurring, but this probability depends on the temperature and diminishes rapidly as the temperature rises.

The magnitude of the Coulomb force depends on the electric charges of the nuclei. The nuclei of heavier elements, which possess more protons, interact with each other more strongly; hence, a higher temperature is required than in the case of lighter nuclei. For this reason, as well as the fact hydrogen is the most abundant element in stars, conversions of hydrogen to helium are the most effective nuclear processes at lower temperatures (of the order of 10^7 °K). These reactions are also responsible for energy production in the Sun.

The combination of four hydrogen nuclei results in one helium nucleus, two positrons, and two neutrinos. The atomic mass of helium, expressed in terms of the mass of the hydrogen atom, is 3.9716, and hence is less than the masses of the hydrogen atoms participating in the reaction; thus the mass loss is $4 - 3.9716 = 0.0284$ which, expressed in grams

$$M = 0.0284 m_H = 4.75 \times 10^{-26} \text{ g}, \qquad (4\text{-}38)$$

is converted into energy. This energy can be calculated from Einstein's law

$$E = mc^2 = 4.27 \times 10^{-5} \text{ erg}. \qquad (4\text{-}39)$$

Part of this energy is released as kinetic energy of the particles produced in the reaction and the rest consists of electromagnetic radiation. Thus, the reaction of the conversion of hydrogen to helium may be written as

$$4_1 H^1 \rightarrow {}_2 He^4 + 2e^+ + 2\nu + \gamma, \qquad (4\text{-}40)$$

where e^+ denotes a positron, ν a neutrino, γ energy radiated during the reaction, the superscripts denote the numbers of nucleons while the subscripts stand for the number of protons in the nucleus. The positrons released in reaction (4-40) are annihilated upon coming into contact with free electrons. The neutrinos, which have an extremely high penetrating power, leave the star. These are the only particles to reach us from the cores of stars. Much hope is now placed on being able to observe the neutrino fluxes in future since they may provide direct information about processes occurring in the cores of stars.

Reaction (4-40) never takes place directly but comes about as the result of a cycle of nuclear reactions.

One such cycle is the proton-proton reaction which proceeds as follows:

$$_1 H^1 + {}_1 H^1 \rightarrow {}_1 H^2 + e^+ + \nu, \qquad (4\text{-}41)$$

$$_1 H^2 + {}_1 H^1 \rightarrow {}_2 He^3 + \gamma, \qquad (4\text{-}42)$$

$$_2 He^3 + {}_2 He^3 \rightarrow {}_2 He^4 + 2 {}_1 H^1. \qquad (4\text{-}43)$$

The proton-proton chain may also end in another way. Namely, instead of reaction (4-43) there may be a cycle of reactions in which nuclei of helium, beryllium and lithium, or of helium, beryllium, and boron are catalysts. The amount of these elements does not change during a cycle, however, and the alternative to (4-43) as an ending to the proton-proton chain may be written briefly as

$$_2 He^3 + {}_1 H^1 + M \rightarrow {}_2 He^4 + e^+ + \nu + M + \gamma, \qquad (4\text{-}44)$$

where M denotes the catalyst nucleus.

Another cycle, which results in reaction (4-40), is the carbon-nitrogen cycle which proceeds as follows:

$$_6 C^{12} + {}_1 H^1 \rightarrow {}_7 N^{13} + \gamma, \qquad (4\text{-}45)$$

$$_7 N^{13} \rightarrow {}_6 C^{13} + e^+ + \nu, \qquad (4\text{-}46)$$

$$_6 C^{13} + {}_1 H^1 \rightarrow {}_7 N^{14} + \gamma, \qquad (4\text{-}47)$$

$$_7\mathrm{N}^{14}+{}_1\mathrm{H}^1 \rightarrow {}_8\mathrm{O}^{15}+\gamma, \tag{4-48}$$

$$_8\mathrm{O}^{15} \rightarrow {}_7\mathrm{N}^{15}+e^++\nu, \tag{4-49}$$

$$_7\mathrm{N}^{15}+{}_1\mathrm{H}^1 \rightarrow {}_6\mathrm{C}^{12}+{}_2\mathrm{He}^4. \tag{4-50}$$

Carbon, nitrogen, and oxygen are catalysts in the carbon-nitrogen cycle. They do take part in the individual reactions, but the amount of these elements remains unchanged as a result of the entire cycle. However, they are necessary for the cycle to take place and hence the rate of the cycle (the amount of energy produced in a unit mass in a unit time) depends on, among other things, the abundance of these elements in the star.

The rate ε of the cycle depends not only on the chemical composition but also on the density ϱ and the temperature T of the gas. At higher temperatures, thermonuclear reactions occur more frequently in the medium, and ε increases with the temperature. Since the carbon-nitrogen cycle reactions occur between nuclei with higher electric charge than in the proton-proton reaction, the rate depends more on the temperature in the case of the carbon cycle than it does in the case of the proton-proton chain. When the rate of energy production in thermonuclear processes is represented by means of the approximative formula

$$\varepsilon = \varepsilon(\varrho, T; X, Y, Z) = \varepsilon^*(X, Y, Z)\varrho T^n \tag{4-51}$$

then at temperatures existing in the centre of the Sun n is somewhat less than 4 for the proton-proton reaction, while for the carbon cycle n is equal to about 19. Because of this temperature-dependence, the proton-proton reaction is more effective at temperatures of less than about 15–20 million degrees, whereas at higher temperatures the carbon cycle is more effective.

Other reactions—apart from those mentioned above—which can take place in a star are those which lead to the synthesis of heavier nuclei: conversion of helium to carbon, carbon to oxygen, oxygen and helium to neon, carbon to magnesium, neon, or sodium, etc. However, a very high temperature is required for these reactions to take place and for that reason in stars similar in structure to the Sun the rate of such reactions is practically zero.

On the basis of laboratory and theoretical investigations, we are in a position to determine the shape of the function $\varepsilon = \varepsilon(\varrho, T; X, Y, Z)$. Knowing the density, the temperature, and the chemical composition, we can calculate the amount of energy produced by every gram of matter in a star in a second.

We can now proceed to compute the flux of energy flowing through a star. Let $L(r)$ denote the amount of energy leaving a sphere $S(r)$ in one second. $L(r)$ must be equal to the amount of energy produced in a second in thermonuclear reactions inside the sphere $S(r)$. Since $\varrho\varepsilon$ ergs of energy are generated in each cm³ of gas in a second,

$$L(r) = \int\limits_{S(r)} \varrho\varepsilon\, dV = 4\pi \int\limits_0^r \varrho\varepsilon r^2 dr. \qquad (4\text{-}52)$$

Differentiating, we can rewrite Eq. (4-52) as

$$\frac{dL(r)}{dr} = 4\pi\varrho(r)\varepsilon r^2. \qquad (4\text{-}53)$$

Section 41   Energy Transport in a Star

Hitherto we have derived four equations of the internal structure of stars: Eqs. (4-18), (4-19), (4-20), and (4-53). They contain five unknown functions: $p(r)$, $\varrho(r)$, $M(r)$, $T(r)$, and $L(r)$. We thus have fewer equations than unknowns. The missing fifth equation will be obtained by considering modes of energy transfer in a star.

Since the thermal conduction of gases is not large inside the star, energy can be transported by convection or radiation. In convection, the gas experiences motion: hotter gas is carried upwards, where it transfers its heat to cooler layers, and once cooled, flows back towards the hotter layers where it is reheated. In this way, energy is conveyed from the hotter lower layers of the star to the upper layers. Where no vertical motion of matter takes place, energy is conveyed by radiation. Emitted in the lower layers, energy flows upwards as electromagnetic radiation, which is scattered, absorbed and re-emitted (but at different wavelengths) by ions and electrons in the successive layers of the star.

Let us consider what conditions must prevail in the star for convective energy transfer, i.e. for vertical motions of matter to be produced and maintained in the star. To this end, let us assume that some element of

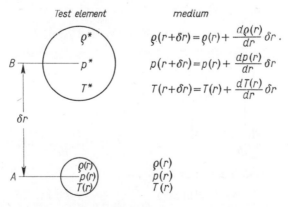

Figure 4-6. Finding the conditions for convection.

mass in layer A at a distance r from the centre of the star is carried upwards through a very small interval δr to layer B (Cf. Fig. 4-6). Conserving the heat contained in it, this element expands since a lower pressure prevails in the medium now surrounding it (in layer B). Our element is assumed to expand adiabatically because we are seeking the condition that energy be transported along with the matter. If now the density of the element is less than that of the surrounding medium, then by Archimedes' principle, this element will continue to move upwards by itself; otherwise, if it were heavier it would drop down to the original position. Thus, the condition for convection to exist is that

$$\varrho^* < \varrho(r+\delta r), \tag{4-54}$$

or, in view of the equality of pressures,

$$p^* = p(r+\delta r), \tag{4-55}$$

that

$$T^* > T(r+\delta r) = T(r) + \frac{dT(r)}{dr}\,\delta r. \tag{4-56}$$

From Eq. (4-56) we have

$$\frac{T^*}{T(r)} > 1 + \frac{d\ln T(r)}{dr}\,\delta r. \tag{4-57}$$

The left-hand side of the inequality (4-57) can be calculated by considering the temperature variations in the given element. Adiabatic transformations in ideal gases are governed by the relation

$$\frac{T^*}{T(r)} = \left(\frac{p^*}{p(r)}\right)^{\frac{\gamma-1}{\gamma}}, \tag{4-58}$$

where γ is the ratio of specific heats

$$\gamma = \frac{c_p}{c_v} \tag{4-59}$$

(c_p is the specific heat at constant pressure, and c_v is the specific heat at constant volume). Equation (4-55) can be used to rewrite Eq. (4-58) as

$$\frac{T^*}{T(r)} = \left[\frac{p(r+\delta r)}{p(r)}\right]^{\frac{\gamma-1}{\gamma}} = \left[\frac{p(r)+\dfrac{dp(r)}{dr}\,\delta r}{p(r)}\right]^{\frac{\gamma-1}{\gamma}}$$

$$= \left[1 + \frac{d\ln p(r)}{dr}\,\delta r\right]^{\frac{\gamma-1}{\gamma}} \approx 1 + \frac{\gamma-1}{\gamma}\,\frac{d\ln p(r)}{dr}\,\delta r. \tag{4-60}$$

Thus, condition (4-57) assumes the form

$$1 + \frac{\gamma-1}{\gamma}\,\frac{d\ln p(r)}{dr}\,\delta r > 1 + \frac{d\ln T(r)}{dr}\,\delta r, \tag{4-61}$$

or

$$\frac{\gamma-1}{\gamma} \frac{d\ln p(r)}{dr} < \frac{d\ln T(r)}{dr}, \tag{4-62}$$

and since $\dfrac{d\ln T(r)}{dr} < 0$ (the temperature decreases with distance from the centre of the star), whereas $(\gamma-1)/\gamma > 0$, therefore

$$\frac{d\ln p(r)}{d\ln T(r)} < \frac{\gamma}{\gamma-1}. \tag{4-63}$$

Inequality (4-63) is a condition for convection motions to exist inside the star. If for any reason such temperature and pressure gradients were to be established in some layer of a star so that inequality (4-63) were satisfied, then strong vertical motions of gas would occur. Rapid mixing of gas across the entire thickness of the layer would ensue. This mixing would cause the temperature gradient to decrease and, hence, the left-hand side of inequality (4-63) to increase. A reduction of the temperature gradient results in the elements of gas moving in the convective layer at a lower velocity, and this means a decrease in the energy flux transported by convection. Convective equilibrium is established when the energy flux transported by convection does not exceed the flux of energy flowing into the lower surface of the convective layer. A gradient of temperature, pressure, and density is then set up in the star. It turns out that even if all the energy reaching the convective layer from the interior were to be transported by convection in that layer, the left-hand side of inequality (4-63) would be not much smaller than the right-hand side. For practical purposes, it is sufficient to assume that the two sides are equal in the convection layer, which means that the adiabatic equation

$$\frac{d\ln p(r)}{d\ln T(r)} = \frac{\gamma}{\gamma-1} \tag{4-64}$$

is satisfied for this layer, or, if use is made of the equation of state, that

$$p(r) = K[\varrho(r)]^{\gamma}, \tag{4-65}$$

where K is a constant.

If inequality (4-63) is not satisfied,

$$\frac{d\ln p(r)}{d\ln T(r)} > \frac{\gamma}{\gamma-1}, \tag{4-66}$$

convection will not develop in the star and the energy is then transported only by radiation. Accordingly, the star is said to be in radiative equilibrium. Since $\gamma = \frac{5}{3}$ for monoatomic gases, the condition for radiative equilibrium can be written as

$$\frac{d\ln p(r)}{d\ln T(r)} > \frac{5}{2}. \tag{4-67}$$

The right-hand side of inequality (4-67) changes, for instance when the gas in the layer under consideration is partially ionized. In that case, partial recombination of gas atoms ensues in the rising element as a result of a drop in temperature during expansion. This process is accompanied by the release of energy. In this way the amount of energy contained in the element increases and this is conducive to convection in the layer. For this reason, the right-hand side of inequality (4-66) grows in layers where the medium is partially ionized. Such a case occurs in the subphotospheric layers of the Sun where hydrogen undergoes ionization. This is the reason why a subphotospheric convection layer comes into being (Cf. Sec. 34).

In order to obtain the missing equation for the structure of stellar interiors, one which holds for layers in radiative equilibrium, we must consider the interaction of the radiation flux with the matter contained in those layers.

Basically speaking, three processes are responsible for absorption of radiation in the interiors of stars. The first of these is further ionization of the ions in the medium by the radiation. When a light quantum absorbs an electron, an ion is knocked out of it. Since hydrogen and helium are completely ionized in the stellar interior, only the ions of heavier elements which retain some electrons in their outer orbits are active in this process. However, the rate of this process also depends on the abundance of hydrogen and helium since these elements (the most plentiful in the star) are the principal suppliers of free electrons which affect the degree of ionization of the heavier elements. The second process under discussion is that of absorption of radiation in the course of free-free transitions of electrons. This happens when a free electron in the field of some ion is accelerated, absorbing a quantum of energy. The third process is that of scattering on free electrons, which results in the direction of the photons of the incident radiation being changed. Important in the surface layers of a star is absorption at wavelengths which could cause atoms to be excited (without being ionized) to higher energy states. The absorption coefficient $\varkappa$ depends on factors which determine the efficiency of the aforementioned processes, that is, on the density, temperature, and chemical composition of the medium. Without going into any detailed discussion of the analytical form of this coefficient, we may write

$$\varkappa = \varkappa(\varrho, T; X, Y, Z). \qquad (4\text{-}68)$$

Let us denote the radiation pressure by $p_r(r)$. By Eq. (4-16), we have

$$\frac{dp_r(r)}{dr} = -g^*(r)\varrho(r), \qquad (4\text{-}69)$$

where $g^*(r)$ is the acceleration imparted to the gas by absorption of radiation. Since acceleration is equal to the amount of momentum gained by 1 gram of gas in the course of 1 second, in order to determine $g^*(r)$ we must calculate the momentum of the radiation absorbed by the gas. Since energy equal to $L(r)$ flows through the surface of the sphere $S(r)$ in 1 second, the energy which flows through each square centimetre of that surface in 1 second is $L(r)/4\pi r^2$. From this we can calculate how much energy is absorbed in 1 second by each gram of matter, namely, $\varkappa L(r)/4\pi r^2$. The momentum of electromagnetic radiation of energy E is E/c (where c is the velocity of light); thus, the momentum which the radiation transfers to each gram of matter in 1 second, or in other words, the acceleration, is

$$g^*(r) = \varkappa \frac{L(r)}{4\pi r^2 c}. \tag{4-70}$$

The spectral distribution of the radiation inside the star can be assumed with great accuracy to be the same as that of blackbody radiation. With this assumption the radiation pressure is determined uniquely by the gas temperature, namely

$$p_r(r) = \tfrac{1}{3}aT^4(r), \tag{4-71}$$

where $a = 7.56 \times 10^{-15} \text{ erg} \cdot \text{cm}^{-3} \cdot \text{deg}^{-4}$.

The final internal-structure equation, which holds in layers where radiative equilibrium exists, thus is of the form

$$\frac{d[\tfrac{1}{3}aT^4(r)]}{dr} = -\frac{\varkappa\varrho(r)L(r)}{4\pi cr^2}. \tag{4-72}$$

Equations (4-65) and (4-72) enter the system of equations for internal stellar structure as alternates. Only one of them is used in a given layer, which one depending on whether or not the pressure and temperature gradients found from Eqs. (4-72) satisfy relation (4-67); if that relation is satisfied, we integrate the stellar model further, using Eq. (4-72); otherwise we employ Eq. (4-65).

Both equations (4-65) and (4-72) can be written in differential form as equations for the temperature derivative. Equations (4-20) and (4-18) can be used to bring Eq. (4-65), after simple manipulations, to the form

$$\frac{dT(r)}{dr} = -\left(\frac{\gamma-1}{\gamma}\right)\frac{GM(r)}{r^2}\frac{\mu}{\mathscr{R}}, \tag{4-73}$$

and Eq. (4-72) can be written as:

$$\frac{dT(r)}{dr} = -\frac{3\varkappa}{4ac}\frac{\varrho(r)L(r)}{4\pi r^2 T^3(r)}. \tag{4-74}$$

Section 42   The Uniqueness of Solutions of the Equations on Internal Stellar Structure

Let us consider the question of the uniqueness of the solutions of the q uations of the internal structure of stars.

The system of these equations consists of four differential equations of the first order:

$$\frac{dp(r)}{dr} = -\frac{GM(r)}{r^2}\,\varrho(r),$$
(4-75)

$$\frac{dM(r)}{dr} = 4\pi\varrho(r)r^2,$$
(4-76)

$$\frac{dL(r)}{dr} = 4\pi\varrho(r)\varepsilon r^2,$$
(4-77)

and (in convective layers)

$$\frac{dT(r)}{dr} = -\left(\frac{\gamma-1}{\gamma}\right)\frac{\mu}{\mathscr{R}}\frac{GM(r)}{r^2},$$

or (in layers in radiative equilibrium)   (4-78)

$$\frac{dT(r)}{dr} = -\frac{3\varkappa}{4ac}\frac{\varrho(r)L(r)}{4\pi r^2 T^3(r)},$$

and one algebraic equation (equation of state):

$$p(r) = f(\varrho(r),\, T(r);\, X,\, Y,\, Z),$$
(4-79)

which in the case of a perfect gas assumes the form

$$p(r) = \frac{\mathscr{R}}{\mu}\,\varrho(r)T(r).$$
(4-79′)

Using Eq. (4-79), we can express the density in terms of the temperature and pressure and thus eliminate it from Eqs. (4-75)–(4-78). Apart from physical constants, the coefficients in these equations are μ, ε, and $\varkappa$. They depend only on the functions $p(r)$ and $T(r)$ [$\varrho(r)$ has already been eliminated by means of Eq. (4-79)] and on the chemical composition X, Y, Z. Thus, the right-hand sides of Eqs. (4-75)–(4-78) are expressed in terms of only the chemical composition and the functions being sought.

Functions $p(r)$, $M(r)$, $L(r)$, and $T(r)$ must satisfy the following boundary conditions at the surface of the star (for $r = R$):

$$p(R) = 0,$$
(4-80)

$$M(R) = \mathfrak{M},$$
(4-81)

$$L(R) = L,$$
(4-82)

$$T(R) = 0.$$
(4-83)

Thus, we have a set of four differential equations (4-75)–(4-78) with four unknown functions $p(r)$, $M(r)$, $L(r)$, and $T(r)$, each of which satisfies one of the four boundary conditions (4-80)–(4-83). This is now sufficient for us to integrate our set of equations and to determine the unknown functions uniquely. These functions will depend on the independent variable r, and the only parameters appearing in them will be the quantities R, $\mathfrak{M}$, L from the boundary conditions and the chemical composition of the star—X, Y, Z, on which the coefficients of Eqs. (4-75)–(4-80) depended. These solutions can be written in the form

$$p = p(r; R, \mathfrak{M}, L, X, Y, Z), \tag{4-84}$$

$$M = M(r; R, \mathfrak{M}, L, X, Y, Z), \tag{4-85}$$

$$L = L(r; R, \mathfrak{M}, L, X, Y, Z), \tag{4-86}$$

$$T = T(r; R, \mathfrak{M}, L, X, Y, Z). \tag{4-87}$$

But for $r = 0$ (for the centre of the star), of course, we must have

$$M(0; R, \mathfrak{M}, L, X, Y, Z) = 0, \tag{4-88}$$

and

$$L(0; R, \mathfrak{M}, L, X, Y, Z) = 0. \tag{4-89}$$

These two boundary conditions [(4-88) and (4-89)] are independent of the conditions at the surface and for that reason—unless further postulated—they might, of course, not be satisfied by solutions which take account only of conditions (4-80)–(4-83). But we now have an excess of boundary conditions in relation to the number of equations and unknowns. Therefore the set of equations will have solutions only for some values of R, $\mathfrak{M}$, L, and Y, Y, Z. Namely, solutions will exist only when those values satisfy conditions (4-88) and (4-89), in which the functions $M(...)$ and $L(...)$ obtained from the solution of the set of equations (4-75)–(4-78) with the boundary conditions (4-80)–(4-83) should be inserted.

In this way, conditions (4-88) and (4-89) are equations associating the radius, mass, brightness, and chemical composition of a star. For stars of identical chemical composition they are the equations of two surfaces in the R, $\mathfrak{M}$, L space. From the fact that we observe stars in nature it follows that these surfaces intersect, that is, that there exist such values of R, $\mathfrak{M}$, and L which satisfy Eqs. (4-88) and (4-89), simultaneously. These surfaces may coincide on some area (then the family of solutions of equations of the internal structure of stars will be a two-parameter family) or will intersect along a curve (or curves); in that case the family of solutions is a one-parameter family. Since the internal-structure equations do not have analytical solutions, we cannot a priori decide which of the two cases occurs in actual fact. A partial solution of this problem can be sought by means of numerical calculations. It would seem that we rather have the second case—the intersection of surfaces specified by Eqs. (4-88) and (4-89) along a curve (or curves) l in the R, $\mathfrak{M}$, L space (only if we adopt such sets of values of R, $\mathfrak{M}$, L which are coordinates of points lying on this curve can we construct a model of the internal stellar structure). Points at which curve l pierces the plane $\mathfrak{M} = \mathfrak{M}_0$ correspond to models of stars of the same mass $\mathfrak{M}_0$. The number of such points depends on the shape of the curve l as specified by Eqs. (4-88) and (4-89). Once again, inasmuch as the analytical forms of these equations are not known, we must resort to numerical calculations. For instance, for $\mathfrak{M} = \mathfrak{M}_\odot$, if the chemical composition is taken to be the same as for the Sun, we obtain at least two different models: a model of the Sun and a model of a white dwarf with the same mass as the Sun. For less massive stars the number of different models of the same mass may be greater: a star built of a perfect gas, a white dwarf, and a neutron star (in the latter case, the nuclei of the atoms of which the star is built are converted to neutrons).

To find the relation between the radius, mass, and brightness of a star (for a given chemical composition), we solve Eqs. (4-88) and (4-89) for R and L, thus obtaining a parametric equation of curve l, in which $\mathfrak{M}$ is the parameter. This process, as we have seen, may not be unique; curve l may have several branches, each of which will be described by another set of equations of the type

$$R = R_i(\mathfrak{M}; X, Y, Z), \qquad (4\text{-}90)$$

and

$$L = L_i(\mathfrak{M}; X, Y, Z), \qquad (4\text{-}91)$$

where the subscripts i are the consecutive numbers of the branches l_i of curve l. Thus, on each of these branches the mass and chemical composition determine R and L; hence, on each branch l_i solutions of Eqs. (4-84)–(4-87) will be determined by the mass and chemical composition:

$$p = p_i(r; \mathfrak{M}; X, Y, Z), \qquad (4\text{-}92)$$

$$M = M_i(r; \mathfrak{M}; X, Y, Z), \qquad (4\text{-}93)$$

$$L = L_i(r; \mathfrak{M}; X, Y, Z), \qquad (4\text{-}94)$$

$$T = T_i(r; \mathfrak{M}; X, Y, Z). \qquad (4\text{-}95)$$

Hence the conclusion is that the models of the internal structure of stars can be arranged in sequences corresponding to the various branches of the curve described by Eqs. (4-90) and (4-91); within these sequences these models are determined only by the mass and the chemical composition. This conclusion has, however, been reached with some assumptions [that the surfaces described by Eqs. (4-88) and (4-89) have no area in common and that the curve l, which is the intersection of these surfaces, has no reactilinear segments perpendicular to the $\mathfrak{M}$ axis] which may be confirmed or refuted only by further numerical calculations.

Calculation of a model of internal structure does not mean that the star described by this model may actually exist. It may be that the star with parameters specified by the model is unstable, that is, that under perturbation of its state it subsequently will continue to change its structure spontaneously, deviating from the state predicted by the model. Such models of internal structure must be rejected [even though they satisfy all Eqs. (4-75)–(4-79) and boundary conditions (4-80)–(4-83), (4-88) and (4-89)].

Section 43 Physical Variable Stars

In previous sections we have discussed stars which did not vary in time. We could not have made this assumption in regard to a group of stars called physical variable stars. The brightness of these stars, their radius, effective temperature, and other parameters do not remain constant but are subject to variations.

For some physical variable stars the dependence of the brightness, radius, and other parameters characterizing the variability of the star is a periodic function of time. Such stars are called regular variables. This group includes cepheids, among others. Variations of brightness are accompanied by the pulsation of these stars; these pulsations have been confirmed by periodic shifts of all lines in the spectrum of a star alternately towards the violet and towards the red, which is evidence of radial motions of the stellar photosphere.

Without discussing the processes responsible for the pulsation of cepheids, we may try to link the period of variation of brightness with other quantities characterizing these stars. If we were to assume that all the features of cepheids (hence, their period $\mathscr{P}$ as well) are uniquely determined by two parameters, e.g. by the gravitational acceleration at the surface of the star, $G\mathfrak{M}/R^2$, and the stellar radius R, we could then seek some simplified relation between $\mathscr{P}$, $G\mathfrak{M}/R^2$, and R. Suppose that this relation can be written as a power function

$$\mathscr{P} = A' \left(\frac{G\mathfrak{M}}{R^2} \right)^{\alpha} R^{\beta}, \tag{4-96}$$

where A' is a dimensionless factor, and α and β are constant exponents. The numerical values of α and β can be found by comparing the dimensions of the left- and right-hand sides of Eq. (4-96). Since $[\mathscr{P}] = \sec$, $[G\mathfrak{M}/R^2] = \text{cm} \cdot \sec^{-2}$, $[R] = \text{cm}$ (where $[f]$ denotes the dimension of f), then by Eq. (4-96)

$$\sec = \text{cm}^{\alpha+\beta}\sec^{-2\alpha}, \tag{4-97}$$

whence

$$\alpha + \beta = 0, \quad -2\alpha = 1. \tag{4-98}$$

Thus

$$\alpha = -\tfrac{1}{2} \quad \text{and} \quad \beta = \tfrac{1}{2}. \tag{4-99}$$

Upon substitution of α and β, Eq. (4-96) becomes

$$\mathscr{P} = A'G^{-\frac{1}{2}}\left(\frac{\mathfrak{M}}{R^3}\right)^{-\frac{1}{2}} = A\bar{\varrho}^{-\frac{1}{2}}, \qquad (4\text{-}100)$$

where A is a constant, while $\bar{\varrho}$ denotes the mean density of the star.

Thus the period of cepheids is inversely proportional to the square root of the mean density. However, the internal structure of the star also has some influence on the value of the proportionality factor A. Consequently, formula (4-100) with a constant value of A could be applied only to a group of cepheids which other sources have shown to be similar in internal structure. Stars which differ considerably in respect to internal structure will be characterized by different values of the coefficient A or, more generally, the relation between the period and the parameters characterizing these stars will be different.

Of particular interest to us is the relation between the period and the luminosity of cepheids. This relationship was discovered observationally by comparing the luminosities and periods of groups of cepheids which were known to be at practically the same distance. The results of this comparison are given in Fig. 4-7.

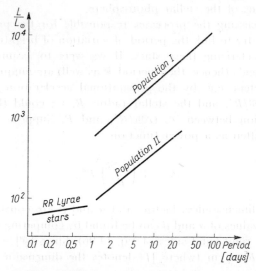

Figure 4-7. The luminosity-period relation for cepheids.

On the basis of this diagram cepheids can be classified as short-period ($\mathscr{P} < 1^d$), also called RR Lyrae stars, and long-period cepheids ($\mathscr{P} > 1^d$) and these, in turn, as stars belonging to population I and II (Cf. Sec. 49). These groups are characterized by different period-luminosity relations.

The period-luminosity relation of cepheids is used frequently to evaluate distance. Knowing the period of a cepheid from observation, we can determine the amount of energy leaving its surface in a unit time and this can serve as a basis for determining the distance (Cf. Sec. 45).

Not all physical variable stars display periodic variations in luminosity. In some, these variations are of an irregular nature and at times are reminiscent of violent explosions. This category includes novae and supernovae. The luminosity of novae increases suddenly (for 1–2 days) by a factor of 10^4–10^6. Upon reaching a maximum, the luminosity of a nova begins to fall off gradually; in general, the brighter a nova is at its maximum, the more rapidly it fades. During and after the explosion the spectrum of the light from nova is usually observed to contain broad lines shifted to the violet and these may be evidence that the outburst is accompanied by the ejection of an outer layer of the star in the form of a shell. Much more violent explosions occur in the case of supernovae. Their maximum brightness is greater than that of the Sun by a factor of the order of 10^8 or more. The explosion of a supernova is accompanied by the release of such enormous energies that it frequently may outshine the entire galaxy in which it appears. Supernovae are regarded in general as the most productive source of primary cosmic radiation. However, they are relatively rare. In our Galaxy, supernova explosions were observed on three occasions in the past thousand years—in 1054, 1572, and 1604. The remnant of the first of these is the Crab nebula which can be observed today as a cloud of gas expanding at the rate of about 1300 km/sec. The age of this nebula, computed from its present size and rate of expansion, has been found to be 900 years, which corresponds to the time elapsed since the supernova explosion.

Pulsars constitute a separate group of physical variable stars. These objects, discovered by radio astronomy at the turn of 1967/68, emit radiation in the form of flashes which are repeated cyclically with a period of 1 second or less (Cf. Fig. 4-8). A characteristic feature of these flashes

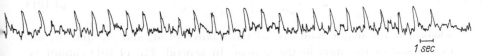

1 sec

Figure 4-8. Series of pulses of radio emission from the pulsar denoted by the symbol CP0808 [After Cole, Pilkington, *Nature*, **219**, 574 (1968)].

is the stability of their period, which increases very slowly indeed. The shape and phase of the flashes changes with the wavelength of the radio radiation at which the observations are made; their amplitudes exhibit a considerable irregularity. In 1969, a pulsar was identified with an optical object—one of the stars in the centre of the Crab nebula; the same star was also found to have pulsations in visible light. The brief period of pulsation of radiation received from pulsars (and the extremely short duration of the flash itself) are indicative of the small size of the pulsars. The most widely accepted hypothesis concerning the structure of pulsars at present treats them as neutron stars which possess powerful magnetic fields and rotate with a period equal to the period of pulsation. On the surface of these stars (according to this hypothesis) is a "sore" through which high-energy particles get into the magnetosphere of the pulsar, where they glow as they are accelerated by the strong magnetic field of the star. Pulsars would in this way supply high-energy particles to the surrounding regions. The coincidence of the positions of the pulsar in the Crab nebula and the supernova of 1054 may be a basis for speculating that pulsars are remnants of supernova explosions.

Section 44   Binary Stars

Eclipsing stars constitute a separate group of variables. These are systems of several (most frequently, two) stars. The variability of the brightness of such a system is due to the components of the system eclipsing each other, not to processes occurring in the stars themselves.

Observations of eclipsing stars may be used to determine the masses of the stars. Indeed, variations in the brightness of the system, and particularly their period, is determined by the motion of the system, which depends on the masses of the components. Let us consider a system consisting of only two stars such that the line-of-sight lies exactly in the plane of motion of the stars. In a system consisting of two bodies the motion is periodic (Cf. Ch. 3) and, therefore, the variations of brightness will also be periodic. Thus, the period of revolution $\mathscr{P}$ can be found from observations of the brightness of the system. To determine the masses of the components, we make use of Kepler's third law

$$\frac{a^3}{\mathscr{P}^2} = \frac{G(m_1+m_2)}{4\pi^2}, \tag{4-101}$$

where a is the major semi-axis of the relative orbit, and m_1 and m_2 are the masses of the stars in the system. In general, Eq. (4-101) cannot be used directly since the major semi-axis a is not known. It is true that if the angular distance α between the stars of a system can be measured when they are furthest apart and if the distance r of the system from the Sun is known, the value of a can be calculated from the formula

$$a = r\alpha. \tag{4-102}$$

However, the value so computed for the major semi-axis of the orbit may have a large error due to the uncertain estimate of the distance r of the system and the error with which the angle α has been measured. A much more accurate method is one based on measuring the radial velocity of the components of the system. This method can be used if we can obtain the spectra of light from both components. From the shift of spectral lines we can find the maximum radial velocities of the components, as well as the radial velocity of the system. The differences between the maximum radial velocities of the components and the radial velocity of the system are equal to the velocities of the components in their orbital motion around a common centre of mass (we shall here assume the motion to be circular). Let us denote the velocities of the components by v_1 and v_2, and the radii of their orbits with respect to the centre of mass of the system by a_1 and a_2. Of course, [Cf. Eqs. (3-29) and (3-30)],

$$\frac{m_2}{m_1} = \frac{a_1}{a_2} = \frac{v_1}{v_2}.$$ (4-103)

Since for circular motion we have

$$\mathscr{P}v_1 = 2\pi a_1,$$ (4-104)

$$\mathscr{P}v_2 = 2\pi a_2,$$ (4-105)

and by the definition of relative motion

$$a = a_1 + a_2,$$ (4-106)

thus

$$a = \frac{\mathscr{P}}{2\pi}(v_1 + v_2).$$ (4-107)

Substituting Eq. (4-107) into Eq. (4-101), we obtain

$$G(m_1 + m_2) = \frac{\mathscr{P}}{2\pi}(v_1 + v_2)^3.$$ (4-108)

Since the right-hand sides of Eqs. (4-103) and (4-108) are known from observations, we can thus determine the masses of both components.

The most advantageous case has been considered here. In general, the orbital plane of a binary system is inclined to the line-of-sight and, moreover, the orbit is not circular. In these cases, the elements of the relative orbit must first be calculated on the basis of an accurate analysis of variations in the brightness of the system over an entire period; and only after Eqs. (4-103) and (4-108) are amended by the corrections stemming from the inclination and the eccentricity of the orbit can the masses of the components be found. Use of binary systems, particularly eclipsing binaries, provides the sole direct, observational method of determining the masses of stars.

Chapter 5 Galactic Structure

POPULATIONS

Section 45 The Scale of Stellar Magnitudes

Brightness and spectral type are the principal physical characteristics of stars.

In astronomy, the observed brightness of a star is expressed in stellar magnitudes. This is a unit based on the old Ptolemaic classification of stars according to their brightness whereby stars visible to the naked-eye were divided into six groups, the brightest-appearing stars being placed in the first magnitude (first-magnitude stars, 1^m) while the faintest were of the sixth magnitude (sixth-magnitude stars, 6^m). As more accurate measurements of stellar illumination received from stars were made, it was found that (a) the ratio of illumination from two stars which differ in brightness by 1^m is constant (does not depend on the brightness of the stars), and (b) the luminous flux from a first-magnitude star is practically 100 times that from a sixth-magnitude star. These two facts serve to define the scale of stellar magnitude now used.

If $\mathcal{E}(m)$ denotes the illumination from a star of apparent magnitude m, then by (a) we have

$$\frac{\mathcal{E}(m)}{\mathcal{E}(m+1)} = a, \tag{5-1}$$

where a is a constant.

Utilizing Eq. (1) and taking (b) into account, we arrive at

$$100 = \frac{\mathcal{E}(1)}{\mathcal{E}(6)} = \frac{\mathcal{E}(1)}{\mathcal{E}(2)} \cdot \frac{\mathcal{E}(2)}{\mathcal{E}(3)} \cdot \frac{\mathcal{E}(3)}{\mathcal{E}(4)} \cdot \frac{\mathcal{E}(4)}{\mathcal{E}(5)} \cdot \frac{\mathcal{E}(5)}{\mathcal{E}(6)} = a^5, \tag{5-2}$$

whence

$$\log a = \tfrac{2}{5} = 0.4. \tag{5-3}$$

The ratio of illuminations from a star of apparent magnitude m and a star of zero magnitude can be computed as follows:

$$\frac{\mathcal{E}(m)}{\mathcal{E}(0)} = \frac{\mathcal{E}(m)}{\mathcal{E}(m-1)} \cdot \frac{\mathcal{E}(m-1)}{\mathcal{E}(m-2)} \cdot \dots \cdot \frac{\mathcal{E}(2)}{\mathcal{E}(1)} \cdot \frac{\mathcal{E}(1)}{\mathcal{E}(0)} = a^{-m}, \tag{5-4}$$

and, consequently,

$$-m\log a = \log \frac{\mathcal{E}(m)}{\mathcal{E}(0)}. \tag{5-5}$$

Employing Eq. (5-3), we obtain

$$m = -2.5\log\frac{\mathscr{E}(m)}{\mathscr{E}(0)} = -2.5\log\mathscr{E}(m)+b. \qquad (5\text{-}6)$$

The zero point b of the scale of stellar magnitudes has been chosen so the scale be in the best possible agreement with the scale used formerly.

The apparent stellar brightness depends not only on the amount of energy emitted by a star but also on the distance of the star from the observer and on the extinction in the interstellar medium. The concept of the absolute brightness of a star is introduced in order to eliminate these effects. The absolute magnitude M of a star is the magnitude the star would have if it were observed from a distance of 10 pc. Since the illumination is inversely proportional to the square of the distance between a source of light and the observer and depends on the optical thickness of the medium between the star and the observer,

$$\mathscr{E}_r = \mathscr{E}_{10}\left(\frac{10}{r}\right)^2 e^{-\tau(r)}, \qquad (5\text{-}7)$$

where r is the distance of the star from the observer, in parsecs, while $\mathscr{E}_r$ and $\mathscr{E}_{10}$ are, respectively, the illumination observed and the illumination at a distance of 10 pc from the star. Since

$$m = -2.5\log\mathscr{E}_r + b$$
$$= -2.5\log\mathscr{E}_{10} - 2.5\log\left(\frac{10}{r}\right)^2 + 2.5\tau(r)\log e + b$$
$$= M + 5\log r - 5 + A(r), \qquad (5\text{-}8)$$

then, knowing the distance r from the star and the interstellar extinction

$$A(r) = 2.5\log e \cdot \tau(r) = 1.085\tau(r), \qquad (5\text{-}9)$$

and the apparent magnitude m, we can calculate the absolute magnitude. Equation (5-8) is frequently used to determine the distance of stars. In that case, we must previously find the absolute (Cf. Sec. 46) and apparent magnitude of the star as well as the interstellar extinction for that star (Cf. Sec. 59).

Section 46   The Spectral Classification of Stars

At the turn of the century, when a considerable number of photographs of the spectra of light from stars had been obtained, the principles of the spectral classification of stars were worked out at the Harvard College Observatory in the U.S.A. Stars are classified by types according to the relative intensities or strengths of the absorption lines and molecular bands occurring in the spectra of these stars (Plate 19). The various types of stars are denoted by the letters

$$O, B, A, F, G, K, M.$$

Each spectral type of stars is subdivided by numbers 0 to 9. Thus, a star of spectral type $F5$ is one with a spectrum midway between a type F spectrum and a type G spectrum.

The temperature, pressure, and chemical composition of the stellar atmosphere are factors that determine the characteristics of a stellar spectrum. Temperature exerts the greatest influence on the appearance of the spectrum. It determines the extent to which the individual elements are ionized and excited, and, hence, the strengths of the corresponding spectral lines. The differences between dwarfs and giants of the same spectral type (i.e. stars with the same photospheric temperature, but of different radii) have become the basis for a two-dimensional classification specifying each star by luminosity class as well as a given spectral type. The differences in brightness between dwarfs and giants of the same spectral type stem from the fact that since the surface brightness of a star is determined by its temperature (hence, is the same for stars in one and the same spectral type) the energy flux L emitted by the star in a second is proportional to the square of the radius of the star (that is, to its surface area). Hence, the absolute brigthness of a giant is much greater than that of a dwarf of the same spectral type. Luminosity classes are denoted by the Roman numerals I, II, III, IV, and V. The differences in the spectra of stars belonging to different luminosity classes are due to the differences in the pressure in the atmospheres of these stars (Plate 20).

The chemical composition of almost all stars is similar and for that reason does not result in any pronounced differentiation of their spectra. Nevertheless, small differences in the abundance of heavy elements, detected by spectroscopic observations, provide interesting information about the origin of stars.

Stars of the highest effective temperatures (about 30,000–40,000°K) are of type O. The spectra of these stars contain the lines of hydrogen, ionized and neutral helium, as well as very weak lines of highly-ionized heavy elements. As we go to type B, the strength of the hydrogen lines increases, the lines of ionized helium disappear, and lines of ionized nitrogen and oxygen make their appearance. In type A, the hydrogen lines attain maximum strength, helium lines no longer appear, but weak lines of metals exist. Type F is characterized by a further increase in the strength of the metal lines. Numerous lines of metals are a characteristic feature in the spectra of type-G stars. The first molecular bands, primarily of C_2, CH, CN, and OH, show up in the spectra of these stars. The Sun is of this type. Molecular bands are evident in type K and the bands of titanium oxide (TiO) stand out among them. These bands became most intensive in the spectra of type-M stars whose effective temperature is about 3000°K.

There is a small group of stars whose spectra, though similar to those of type-K and type-M stars, do not have the titanium oxide band. Some of them do have the C_2 band and they are classified as type-R and -N stars, while the others display the presence of zirconium oxide ZrO and technetium; the latter are grouped in the spectral type S.

The spectral types also differ as to how the intensity of the radiation is distributed in the continuous spectrum. As we pass from type O to type M, the maximum of the intensity in the continuous spectrum shifts from the violet towards the red. The ratio of the radiation intensities of stars in two colours is

$$\frac{I(\lambda_1)}{I(\lambda_2)} = \frac{\mathscr{E}_{10}(\lambda_1)}{\mathscr{E}_{10}(\lambda_2)} \tag{5-10}$$

[where $I(\lambda_1)$ and $I(\lambda_2)$ denote the radiation intensities of the star in question in the spectral regions in the vicinity of wavelengths λ_1 and λ_2, respectively; the size of these spectral regions is determined by the width of the transmission bands of the filters used in the photometer when the star was observed]. This ratio may serve to determine the temperature of the atmosphere of a star and, hence, indirectly also to determine its spectral class. This ratio, expressed in stellar magnitudes, is called the colour index

$$M(\lambda_1)-M(\lambda_2) = -2.5\log\frac{I(\lambda_1)}{I(\lambda_2)}. \tag{5-11}$$

Knowledge of the colour index may thus serve to determine the spectral type of a star. In practice, instead of the spectral type we frequently give the colour index (for instance, the difference between the absolute brightness in blue and yellow, B–V) or simply the temperature of the atmosphere.

A star is assigned to a particular luminosity class within a given spectral type by estimating the ratio of the intensities of the appropriate pairs of spectral lines. There are six luminosity classes: class Ia comprises the brightest supergiants which are characterized by enormous size, class Ib includes the less bright supergiants, class II consists of bright giants, class III of giants, class IV of subgiants, and class V of dwarfs (Fig. 5-1).

The absolute brightness of stars belonging to a particular spectral type and luminosity class may be determined from calibration based on the trigonometric parallax (Cf. Sec. 15) of near stars. Equation (2-1) of Ch. 2 allows us to calculate the distance of stars which are not too far from the Sun, Knowing their observed brightness, we find their absolute brightness by Eq. (5-8) from the previous section. Observations of the

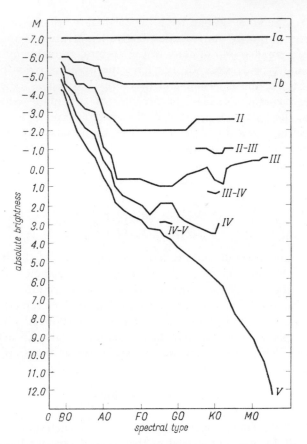

Figure 5-1. Two-dimensional spectral classification [After Bok and Bok, *The Milky Way*, Harvard University Press, Cambridge, Mass., 1957].

spectra of their light serve to classify each of these stars in a particular spectral type and luminosity class. In this way, within the individual spectral types and luminosity classes we have groups of stars (near stars) for which spectral classification and the absolute brightness have been determined independently. If the relation between the absolute brightness of stars and their spectral types and luminosity classes obtained in this way is extrapolated to all observed stars, we can determine the absolute brightness of stars from their spectral classification. Now if we employ Eq. (5-8), we are in a position to compute the distance of the star in question [the estimation of the magnitude of interstellar extinction $A(r)$ will be discussed in the next chapter]. This method of determining the distances of stars is known as the method of spectroscopic parallaxes.

Section 47   The H–R Diagram

In Sec. 42 we found that conditions (4-88) and (4-89) may be expected to result in there being a number of sequences of models for the internal structure of stars such that within each of these sequences the mass and chemical composition determine the stellar model. If the chemical composition of stars belonging to a given sequence were assumed to be the same, then all the parameters characterizing the stars in that group would be functions of only the mass. In particular, the absolute brightness M of these stars and their effective temperature T_e would be determined by the masses of the stars

$$M_e = M_e(\mathfrak{M}),\qquad(5\text{-}12)$$

and

$$T_e = T_e(\mathfrak{M}).\qquad(5\text{-}13)$$

Verification of this supposition could be sought by comparison with observations. Namely, if we were to construct a diagram plotting the effective temperature against the absolute brightness of stars, Eqs. (5-12) and (5-13) would be parametric equations of a curve on which all points corresponding to the stars of a given group would lie (Fig. 5-2).

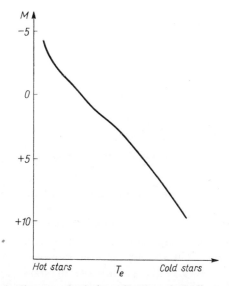

Figure 5-2. Schematic diagram of relations (5-12) and (5-13).

Diagrams of this kind were constructed for the first time in 1905–1913 by Hertzsprung and Russel. Hence, diagrams of absolute magnitude vs. spectral type are frequently called Hertzsprung–Russel (H–R) diagrams. Figure 5-3 is an H–R diagram on which the number of points marked

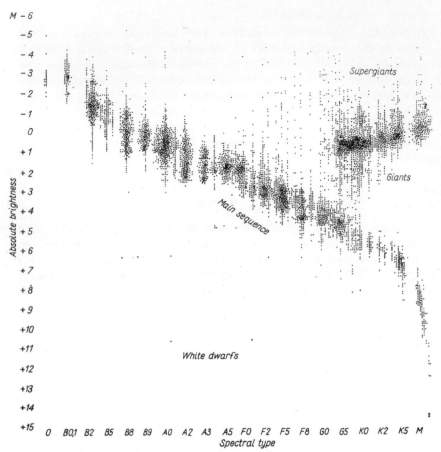

Figure 5-3. H–R diagram for all observed stars [After Gyllenberg, Lund Observatory].

is proportional to the number of observed stars of the corresponding type and magnitude.

The most obvious feature of the diagram is that there is a certain privileged curve which runs diagonally across the figure from the top left corner to the bottom right corner. A considerable numbers of stars is grouped along that curve. This assemblage of stars is called the main sequence. Apart from the main sequence, there is a substantial number of bright type-G and type-K stars. These stars, having the same effective temperatures as main-sequence dwarfs of these types, must be much larger than those dwarfs. The brightest of them are the supergiants, and beneath them in Fig. 5-3 are giants and subgiants. Several points below the main sequence represent white dwarfs, stars of extremely small radii.

Figure 5-3 does not fully convey the actual distribution of stars in the H–R diagram. We observe only the brightest of the remote stars since the faintest are beyond the range of our instruments. In order to obviate this undesirable selection effect, it is necessary to confine ourselves to stars in the immediate vicinity of the Sun. Then, with great probability we can say that we observe all the stars which appear there (Fig. 5-4).

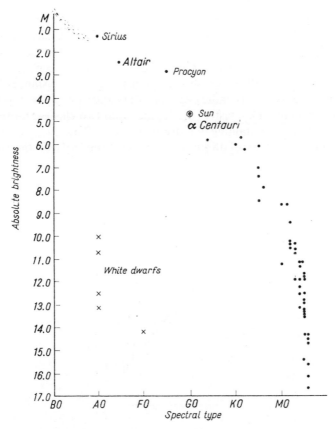

Figure 5-4. H–R diagram for stars not more than 5 pc from Sun [After Bok and Bok, *The Milky Way*, Harvard University Press, Cambridge, Mass., 1957].

Of the 56 stars in the immediate vicinity of the Sun, 51 are main-sequence stars, 5 are white dwarfs, and not one is a giant. The conclusions drawn from Fig. 5-4 are valid only for the neighbourhood of the Sun and we have no right to extend them to any arbitrary region of the Galaxy. The percentage abundance of stars of various spectral types may be different in other regions of the Galaxy.

The occurrence of stars beyond the main sequence indicates that their chemical composition must differ from that of main-sequence stars (major differences in chemical composition can occur only in the cores of these stars). Otherwise, the equilibrium conditions discussed in Ch. 4 are not satisfied in them.

Section 48   Star Clusters

Interesting conclusions can be drawn from H–R diagrams plotted for aggregations of stars which, we have reason to believe, have a common origin. Clusters, systems consisting of many stars situated close together, are natural aggregations of this type. The distances between stars belonging to clusters are small, much shorter than the average distances between stars in the Galaxy; this indicates that stars did not come together by chance to form clusters. Clusters are divided into two classes: those known as galactic clusters containing hundreds of stars (Plate 21), and globular clusters containing tens of thousands or even hundreds of thousands of stars (Plate 22).

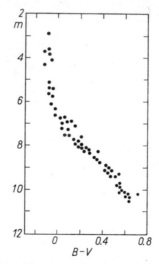

Figure 5-5. H–R diagram for Pleiades. The apparent magnitude in yellow light is laid off along the ordinate axis and the $B-V$ colour index along the abscissa axis [After Johnson and Morgan, *Astrophys. Journ.* **117**, 313 (1953)].

Figure 5-5 shows the H–R diagram for a typical galactic cluster. It is a striking fact that the stars of this cluster fall along one line in the H–R diagram. This is evidence that the cluster is not some random assemblage of stars, and suggests that the stars belonging to it possess some physical features in common. The simplest supposition is that the stars in the cluster are of the same age. If this supposition were true—i.e. that all the stars had come into being at the same time—their chemical composition at the time of origin should have been identical, the same as the composition of the matter out of which the cluster was formed. The feature differentiating the newly-created stars would have been their mass; thus we could expect that on the H–R diagram they would fall in a line which we shall call the zero-age main sequence for the given cluster. Of course, the characteristics of stars could change during evolution and those stars which evolve more rapidly could leave the zero-age main sequence. This would result in the main sequence of the cluster changing continuously, at least for that part on which the fast-evolving stars are located.

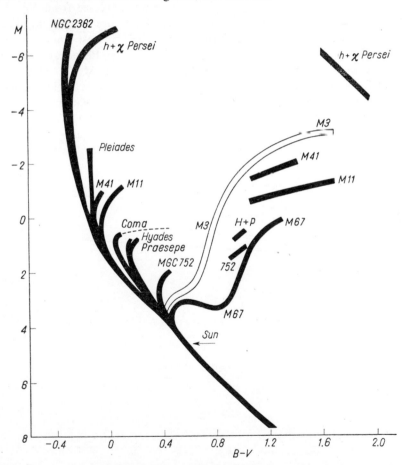

Figure 5-6. A composite H–R diagram for several galactic clusters (heavy lines). and one globular cluster [After Sandage, *Stellar Populations*, Ed. by O'Connell, Vatican Observatory, 1958].

We are unable to trace the changes in the position of the main sequence of a single cluster since such changes occur on a time scale many times that of the period in which regular observations of clusters have been made. We must confine ourselves to compiling H–R diagrams for several galactic clusters and to interpreting the differences in these diagrams as the result of a difference in age (Fig. 5-6).

A characteristic feature of this figure is that the diagrams of the individual clusters deflect to the right in the parts corresponding to the most luminous stars whereas the main sequences for the fainter stars have a common position. This indicates that the most luminous, and hence most massive stars, leave the main sequence most quickly and move to the right on the H–R diagram. At the same time, we see from Fig. 5-6 that the deviation from the original main sequence comes in different places for the various clusters. In some clusters, only the brightest stars have left the zero-age main sequence (e.g. h and χ Persei, the Pleiades), while in others the deviation comes for less massive stars (e.g. M 67). This gives grounds for supposing that the M 67 cluster is older (the evolution of stars belonging to this cluster is more advanced) than the Pleiades. Thus, the position of the point at which deviation of the H–R diagram from the zero-age main sequence begins may serve to determine the age of the cluster. Figure 5-7 is the H–R diagram of one of the oldest galactic clusters, M 67.

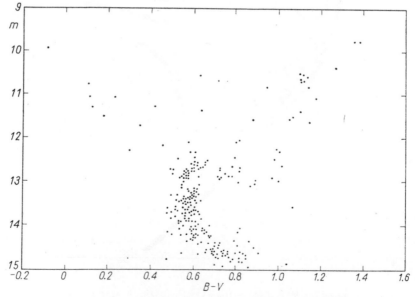

Figure 5-7. The H–R diagram for the cluster M 67 [After Johnson and Sandage, *Astrophys. Journ.* **121**, 616 (1955)].

The H–R diagrams of globular clusters (Fig. 5-8) are similar in character. The weak stars of this cluster have not yet left the main sequence, while the brighter stars lie along a line passing through the region of giants and supergiants. These characteristic features are repeated on the H–R diagrams of other globular clusters.

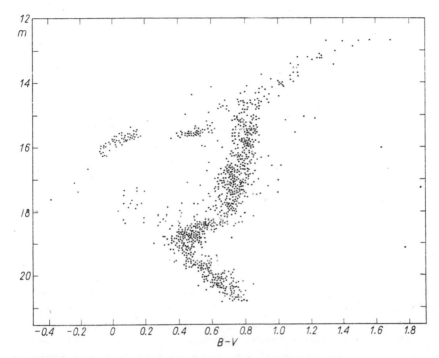

Figure 5-8. The H–R diagram for globular cluster M 3 [After Johnson and Sandage, *Astrophys. Journ.* **124**, 379 (1956)].

The similarity of the H–R diagrams of globular clusters and the oldest galactic clusters suggests that galactic clusters are in general younger than the globular ones. Bear in mind, however, that this is based on the assumption that the differences in the H–R diagrams can be attributed to the stars being at different stages of evolution and that at the time of their origin, the stars in all clusters were aligned in more or less the same fashion on the H–R diagram. To confirm these assumptions, we must refer to other estimates of the age of clusters, estimates that are independent of those given above.

Important information about the age of clusters can be provided by an estimate of their permanency. Stars belonging to a cluster are bound together by mutual gravitational forces. The smaller the radius of the cluster and the more numerous the stars in the cluster, the stronger the gravitational interaction between the stars. Each pair of stars passing each other exchange momentum and mechanical energy, as is the case with colliding gas molecules. In consequence, the distribution of the velocity of stars in a cluster tends to a Maxwellian distribution (Fig. 5-9).

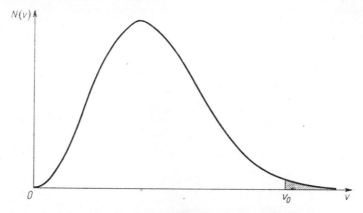

Figure 5-9. Maxwell velocity distribution. $N(v)$ is the number of stars with velocity v.

Inasmuch as a Maxwellian distribution of velocity is established, a number of stars attain velocities in excess of the velocity v_0 sufficient to overcome the gravitational attraction of the other stars; these stars leave the cluster. Encounters which continue to occur within the cluster result in another group of stars acquiring velocities greater than v_0. This process steadily reduces the number of stars in the cluster; the cluster breaks up. The rate at which this happens depends on the relaxation time, i.e. the period of time it takes a Maxwellian distribution to be established in the cluster (Table 5-1).

Once the velocities of the stars in the cluster take on a Maxwellian distribution, some 1% of the total number of stars are moving at velocities

TABLE 5-1

Relaxation Time and Disintegration of Clusters

Type of Cluster	Mass $(\mathfrak{M}_\odot = 1)$	Radius (pc)	Relaxation Time (years)	Disintegration (years)
Globular clusters	10^6	15–20	10^{10}	10^{12}
Pleiades	400	3	3×10^7	3×10^9
Small open clusters	50	1	8×10^6	8×10^8

greater than v_0 and thus the time the cluster takes to break up is longer than the relaxation time by a factor of about 100. For clusters of large radius and irregular shape, the lifetime is even shorter since their breakup is also caused by the tidal gravitational forces of the entire Galaxy; we had no need to take these forces into account in the case of regular, dense clusters.

Extremely unstable assemblages are called associations of stars. They consist of about a hundred stars each. Measurements of the velocities of stars in associations indicate that they disintegrate within 10^7 years. Thus, associations and hence their constituent stars, must be young and must have been of recent origin. This is an obvious proof that the process of the birth of stars is taking place at present.

The data in Table 5-1 show that galactic clusters must be young, their age not exceeding several thousand million years whereas globular clusters may be much older systems. This is in accordance with the previous conclusions concerning the age of clusters, drawn from comparison of their H–R diagrams.

Section 40   Populations

Let us return to Fig. 5-6 which shows the H–R diagrams for clusters M 3 and M 67. One of these, M 67, is an old galactic cluster while the other, M 3, is a globular cluster. Even though the two clusters leave the main sequence at points close to each other on the H–R diagrams, the other parts of these diagrams in the region of the giants differ from each other considerably. Of course, if the stars in both clusters had the same chemical composition at the time of origin, they should evolve identically and the H–R diagrams for both clusters should coincide, or at least lie close to each other. On the basis of this, it may be concluded that the member stars of these clusters had different initial chemical compositions.

TABLE 5-2

Stellar Populations

Population	Typical Components	Abundance of Heavy Elements (%)
Young population I	Young open clusters, O and B stars, interstellar matter	4
Intermediate population I	A and F stars, open clusters, red super-giants	3
Old population I	Main-sequence stars and G and K giants	2
Mild population II	White dwarfs, many classes of variables	1
Extreme population II	Globular clusters, subdwarfs	0.3

This conclusion may also be derived at from observations which confirm that the atmospheres of member stars of globular and galactic clusters differ in chemical composition.

Thus, we can divide all stars in the Galaxy into two groups, two populations. Stars belonging to galactic clusters are characteristic stars of population I, while those in globular clusters are typical of population II. Such a classification is highly simplified, of course. At present, stars are also classified into five groups whose characteristics are given in Table 5-2.

STELLAR EVOLUTION

Section 50   The Theoretical Foundations

The purpose of our discussion will be to provide an answer to the question of what causes the differences in the H–R diagrams for stars of populations I and II, to explain the differences in the chemical composition of their atmospheres, and, finally, to present the tracks of stellar evolution and the transformations of stellar matter during the life of a star.

Our considerations start by following a theoretical model of a star which changes as a result of transformations occurring inside the star. Thus, the parameters of the star–brightness, effective temperature, and spectral type–also vary. This causes the star to be displaced on the H–R diagram. The line along which a point characterizing the current state of a star moves on the H–R diagram is called the evolutionary track. The validity of hypotheses about evolutionary processes taking place in stellar interiors can be tested by comparing the predicted distribution of stars on the H–R diagram with the actual distribution. Thus, if we take a group of stars which we have reason to believe to be of the same age (e.g. they belong to one cluster), we can trace how the H–R diagram changes with time by using some hypothesis concerning the evolutionary changes occurring in those stars. The curve along which the stars are aligned on the H–R diagram at a given time after their birth is called a time line. The fact that one of the theoretical time lines coincides with the H–R diagram made for the given cluster on the basis of observations is an argument for the validity of the hypotheses adopted in making the theoretical stellar model and may serve to determine the age of the cluster.

A basic condition for accurately tracing the evolutionary track is to have an exact model of the stellar structure throughout the life of the star. Unfortunately, our knowledge of the structure of stars in some stages of evolution is inadequate for that purpose at present, and, consequently, the theory given below is somewhat sketchy in some points. A general opinion on the evolution of stars from their birth to their death has, however, grown out of many theoretical results, confirmed by observations.

Section 51   Phase I—The Star Before Reaching the Main
              Sequence

The only known material out of which a star may be formed is the
matter scattered throughout interstellar space (Cf. Ch. 6). As a result of
factors which cause matter to become comparatively dense here and there
in the interstellar medium, condensations begin to form in which the gravitational forces exceed the expansive action of the pressure. Such condensations begin to shrink under the influence of their own gravitational field
and the density in them grows increasingly. A mass of gas contracting in
this way can be regarded as a star in its first evolutionary phase, the phase
of formation. During the contraction the gravitational energy of the star
decreases, becoming converted into thermal energy and thus causing the
temperature to rise. At the same time, the star loses a fraction of its energy
through radiation.

To determine what fraction of the gravitational energy E_G is expended
on increasing the thermal energy E_T during contraction and what fraction
E_R is radiated, let us resort to the following reasoning.

We may assume that at the initial instant, when it is on the verge of
forming out of the gas cloud, the star has a gravitational energy of

$$E_{G0} = 0. \tag{5-14}$$

Indeed, the cloud is then large, and the gravitational interaction between
its parts is insignificant. The thermal energy of the cloud may also be
neglected in comparison with the thermal energy of the star; the temperature of 100°K (of the interstellar gas) is many orders of magnitude smaller
than the temperature in the stellar interior. Thus,

$$E_{T0} = 0. \tag{5-15}$$

Since stellar radiation has not yet commenced,

$$E_{R0} = 0, \tag{5-16}$$

where E_R is the energy radiated by the star from the beginning of contraction. Thus, the total energy

$$E_{G0} + E_{T0} + E_{R0} = 0. \tag{5-17}$$

Since the total energy is zero at the initial instant, it must also be equal
to zero at any other instant, including the one when the contraction ceases
and the star reaches the main sequence, whence

$$E_G + E_T + E_R = 0. \tag{5-18}$$

When the star is on the main sequence, contraction ceases and the conditions of dynamic equilibrium (the star is stationary) are satisfied in the
stellar interior. The relation between the gravitational energy E_G and the
thermal energy E_T in a stationary star can be obtained by using Eq. (4-18).

The thermal energy, that is the energy of the thermal motions of the gas molecules (or the particles if the gas is ionized) in 1 cm³, is given by the formula

$$e_T = \tfrac{1}{2}Nm\overline{v^2}, \tag{5-19}$$

where N is the number of molecules per cm³, m is the mass of one molecule, and $\overline{v^2}$ is the mean-square velocity of the molecules. The pressure p is equal to the force with which the gas molecules act on an area of 1 cm². If we were to put a wall 1 cm² in area at some point, the molecules impinging on it would rebound elastically. If the velocity component perpendicular to the wall is denoted by w, the number of molecules striking the wall in 1 second is $\tfrac{1}{2}Nw$ (half the molecules move towards the wall, and half in the opposite direction). During the rebound the momentum of each molecule changes by $2mw$; hence the total change in momentum is

$$\tfrac{1}{2}Nw \cdot 2mw = Nmw^2. \tag{5-20}$$

If we take account of the fact that the molecules have different velocities, we should insert the mean value of w^2 in Eq. (5-20). Since the directions of the molecule velocities have an isotropic distribution, therefore

$$\overline{w^2} = \tfrac{1}{3}\overline{v^2}. \tag{5-21}$$

Thus, the pressure is

$$p = \tfrac{1}{3}Nm\overline{v^2} = \tfrac{2}{3}e_T. \tag{5-22}$$

The total thermal energy of the star is obtained by integrating e_T over the entire volume of the star

$$E_T = \int_0^R e_T 4\pi r^2 dr = \tfrac{3}{2}\int_0^R p4\pi r^2 dr = [\tfrac{1}{2}p4\pi r^3]_{r=0}^{r=R} - \tfrac{1}{2}\int_0^R \frac{dp}{dr} 4\pi r^3 dr$$

$$= -\tfrac{1}{2}\int_0^R \frac{dp}{dr} 4\pi r^3 dr, \tag{5-23}$$

where

$$[\tfrac{1}{2}p4\pi r^3]_{r=0}^{r=R} = 0 \tag{5-24}$$

($p = 0$ at the stellar surface, whereas at the centre $r^3 = 0$).

Using Eq. (4-18), we have

$$E_T = -\tfrac{1}{2}\int_0^R \frac{dp}{dr} 4\pi r^3 dr = \tfrac{1}{2}\int_0^R \frac{GM(r)}{r} \varrho 4\pi r^2 dr. \tag{5-25}$$

The last integral is the potential energy of the star, but with opposite sign:

$$E_G = -\int_0^R \frac{GM(r)}{r} \varrho(r)4\pi r^2 dr = -\int_0^{\mathfrak{M}} \frac{GM(r)}{r} dM(r). \tag{5-26}$$

Thus, by Eq. (5-25) we have

$$E_T = -\tfrac{1}{2}E_G.$$ (5-27)

In this way we have proved the theorem:

The gravitational energy in a gaseous system in dynamic equilibrium is twice the thermal energy, but of opposite sign.

Applying this to a star which has just reached the main sequence, we can use Eq. (5-18) to calculate the amount of energy radiated by the star during the stage of contraction:

$$E_R = -E_G - E_T = -\tfrac{1}{2}E_G = E_T.$$ (5-28)

Once we know the gravitational or thermal energy of a star on the main sequence we can compute the amount of energy radiated by that star in the formation phase.

The total thermal energy of the Sun is about 5×10^{48} ergs. An equal amount of energy had to be radiated by the Sun up to the time it reached the main sequence. Since the Sun radiates energy at the rate of $3.86 \times \times 10^{33}$ ergs per second, if we assume that the rate of radiation was the same during contraction, we can find the lifetime of the Sun in the formation phase

$$t = \frac{5 \times 10^{48}}{3.86 \times 10^{33}} \sec = 1.3 \times 10^{15} \sec \approx 4 \times 10^7 \text{ years}.$$ (5-29)

In actual fact, this time is longer because as contraction proceeds a star changes its luminosity (Cf. Fig. 5-10) and calculations yield a value of a fifty million years.

The time a star requires to reach the main sequence depends on its mass. More massive stars contract more quickly. Type $B0$ stars, for instance, reach the main sequence in only 10^5 years.

As the density in a star increases, so does its temperature. The rise in effective temperature causes the star to move to the left on the H–R

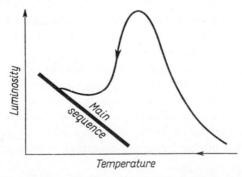

Figure 5-10. The evolutionary track of a star before reaching the main sequence.

diagram. It reaches the main sequence by passing through the region occupied on the H–R diagram by red giants, subgiants, or red dwarfs (Cf. Fig. 5-10), depending on its mass. A steady rise of temperature in the stellar interior creates conditions conducive to nuclear reactions. When conversion of hydrogen to helium begins in the star, further contraction ceases owing to a rise in temperature and pressure; dynamic equilibrium is attained in the star. The star ends the first stage of its life and becomes a member of the main sequence.

Section 52   Phase II—The Star on the Main Sequence

Once stars have reached the main sequence, they continue to change their position on the H–R diagram, that is, their brightness and spectral type keep on changing. These changes may be due to changes either in the mass or the chemical composition of the stars.

The mass of a star could increase through the capture of interstellar matter. This mechanism of mass accretion, however, is highly ineffective because of the high velocities of the stars relative to the gas clouds and the low densities of interstellar matter.

Loss of mass could occur in two ways:

1) ejection of gas from the stellar atmosphere,

2) electromagnetic radiation.

Let us evaluate the efficiency of these processes of mass loss in the case of the Sun. The rate of mass outflow from the Sun could be evaluated from observations of the "solar wind". All measurements give a value of the order of 10^8 particles per cm^2 per sec at a distance of one astronomical unit from the Sun. Thus, the amount of matter leaving the Sun can be evaluated from the intensity of the solar wind to be 5×10^{11} g/sec. The mass lost through electromagnetic radiation can be found from the formula

$$m = \frac{L_\odot}{c^2} = \frac{3.82 \times 10^{33}}{9 \times 10^{20}} \text{ g/sec} = 4 \times 10^{12} \text{ g/sec}. \qquad (5\text{-}30)$$

Thus, the Sun loses no more than 5×10^{12} g in a second. The time required for the Sun to reduce its mass by 1 per cent is of the order of 10^{11} years. This is longer than the age of the Galaxy. We see, therefore, that such a tiny loss of mass cannot explain the evolutionary changes occurring in stars similar to the Sun in structure. A change in the chemical composition in stellar interiors must, therefore, be the determining factor in the evolution of stars. This does not mean, of course, that mass loss cannot be an important evolutionary factor in certain stages in the life of a star; instead, it merely means that nuclear processes occurring in stars are the key factor in evolution.

From the time that nuclear processes "ignite" in the interior of a star, hydrogen is continuously converted to helium. The mean hydrogen abundance $\overline{X}$ in a star decreases while the helium abundance $\overline{Y}$ increases. At its birth, a star has a homogeneous chemical composition throughout its interior, that of the interstellar matter out of which it was formed. In the course of evolution, helium is produced in the central regions of the star where the temperature is high enough for nuclear processes to take place. The evolutionary track of a star depends on what fraction of the hydrogen takes part in this "burn-out". In the case of stars in radiative equilibrium, in which matter does not undergo mixing, the nuclear processes lead to hydrogen depletion only in the core of the star whereas the outer parts retain their original chemical composition. On the contrary, if we were to imagine the model of a star in which convection occurs throughout the entire volume, from the core to the surface, the helium produced would be carried outwards while new portions of hydrogen would flow continuously to the core. As a result, all the hydrogen from the entire volume of the star would be completely depleted, with an almost homogeneous chemical composition being retained. The evolutionary tracks would be different in the two cases, of course. Figure 5-11 shows the evolutionary tracks of

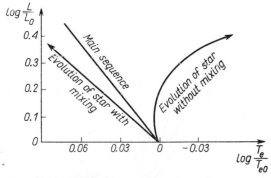

Fig. 5-11. Comparison of the evolutionary tracks of stars with homogeneous and nonhomogeneous chemical composition. L_0 and T_0 are the initial magnitude and effective temperature of the star.

two stars with identical chemical composition at the time of their birth; in one of these stars, the hydrogen only in the core has been burned out, whereas in the other a homogeneous chemical composition is maintained because of convection. Comparison of Fig. 5-11 with the H–R diagram for clusters indicates that only an evolutionary model with depletion of hydrogen in the core corresponds to stars moving to the right of the main sequence as observed.

The remarks above may serve to determine evolutionary tracks. As soon as a star reaches the main sequence, its density and pressure distribution becomes established and does not undergo any major variations in the initial stages of evolution. In particular, the value of the ratio of pressure to density at the centre of the star may then be treated as approximately constant

$$p_c/\varrho_c \approx \text{const.} \qquad (5\text{-}31)$$

The central temperature of the star can be determined from the ideal gas equation

$$T_c = \mu_c \mathscr{R}^{-1} \frac{p_c}{\varrho_c}. \qquad (5\text{-}32)$$

As the hydrogen is converted to helium, the mean molecular mass of matter in the stellar core increases

$$\mu_c = \frac{1}{2X + \frac{3}{4}Y + \frac{1}{2}Z} = \frac{1}{\frac{3}{4} + \frac{5}{4}X - \frac{1}{4}Z}. \qquad (5\text{-}33)$$

A change in μ_c leads in the first place to a rise of temperature. Since the rate of nuclear processes depends strongly on the temperature, the amount of energy produced increases and the star becomes brighter and brighter.

The mass of the star exerts the decisive influence on the rate of evolution. The temperature in the interiors of massive stars attains higher values and, consequently, the conversion of hydrogen to helium proceeds more

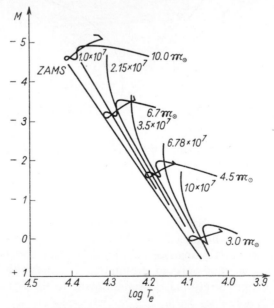

Figure 5-12. Evolutionary tracks for hydrogen-burning models of 3.0, 4.5, 6.7, and 10.0 $\mathfrak{M}_\odot$. Vertical curves—time lines (labelled with cluster age in years); *ZAMS*—zero-age main sequence [After E. Simpson *et al.*, *Astrophys. Journ.* **159**, 896 (1970)].

rapidly and the hydrogen is exhausted sooner. As a result, stars of large masses leave the main sequence earlier than do less massive stars. Time lines for stars of masses from $2.5\mathfrak{M}_\odot$ to $5.6\mathfrak{M}_\odot$ are plotted in Fig. 5-12. These lines have the same characteristic shape as the H–R diagrams for galactic clusters. The most massive members of galactic clusters have already left the main sequence while the less massive are still in the process of burning the hydrogen in their cores.

Section 53   Phase III—The Star with Helium Core

The moment that the hydrogen in the stellar core is completely depleted, the star enters the third stage of its evolution. The evolutionary track in this stage depends on the mass of the star in an important manner (Fig. 5-13). When the hydrogen is exhausted in the central regions, nuclear processes

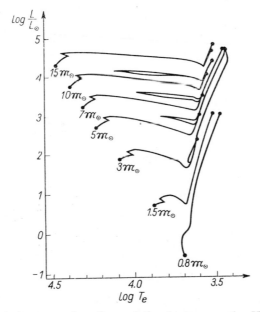

Figure 5-13. Evolutionary tracks of population-I stars on the H–R diagram. Dots indicate the position of the homogeneous main sequence models and the position of the models at the times of helium and carbon ignition in their cores [After B. Paczyński, *Acta Astron.* **20**, 50 (1970)].

cease there and energy production shifts to a thin layer surrounding the core composed mainly of helium, with a slight admixture of heavier elements. The nuclear reactions which maintained the temperature of the central regions at a level ensuring dynamical equilibrium of the star have stopped taking place in the helium core and the result is that the core begins to shrink. This process is accompanied by a development of the envelope and growth of the stellar radius.

In massive stars, the core continues to contract until the temperature in it ignites reactions whereby helium is converted into heavy elements. The appearance of new sources of energy causes a rapid growth of the star which soon becomes a red giant.

Less massive stars, of masses not much more than that of the Sun, evolve in a different manner. Even before the hydrogen has been completely depleted, the cores of such stars possess a very high density. A slight contraction of the helium core that is produced leads to a state in which the gas ceases to have the properties of an ideal gas. The helium core, or at least its central parts, become degenerate. Once degeneracy of helium appears in the core, the pressure increases rapidly and dynamical equilibrium is attained with a slight rise in temperature, which is insufficient

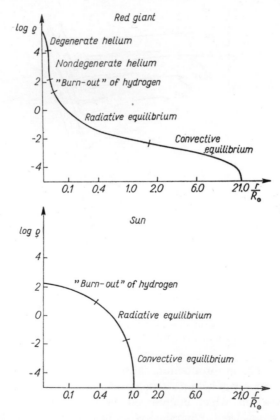

Figure 5-14. Density distribution inside a red giant and a main sequence star of similar mass.

for touching off helium conversions. The model of the star which is thus established consists of an isothermal helium core surrounded by a thin layer in which hydrogen is "burned" and an extended envelope in radiative equilibrium. An extended convective layer (Fig. 5-14) builds up in the outer layers. The star has a much larger radius during this time than in the main-sequence stage. As time passes, the layer where the hydrogen burning occurs moves outwardly and the mass of the helium core increases. The star moves vertically to the right on the H–R diagram, along the sub-giant branch to the region of red giants:

The evolutionary track during this period depends strongly on the initial abundances of heavy elements in the star. Whereas the main sequences for population-I and -II stars differ from each other by no more than $0^m.1$, more pronounced differences appear between the populations once they have left the main sequence (Cf. Fig. 5-15 and compare with Fig. 5-6).

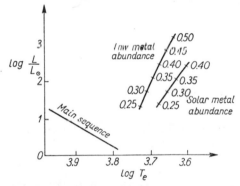

Figure 5-15. Evolutionary tracks of population-I and -II stars. The numbers indicate what fraction of the mass is contained in the helium core [After Martin Schwarzschild, *Structure and Evolution of the Stars* (copyright (c) 1958 by Princeton University Press); reprinted by permission of Princeton University Press].

The rate of evolution along the red giant branch depends on the mass of the star. Figure 5-16 shows the plots of theoretical evolutionary tracks calculated for three stars of only slightly differing masses, lying in the interval between $1.0\mathfrak{M}_\odot$ and $1.2\mathfrak{M}_\odot$. The heavy line corresponds to an age of 10^{10} years for the stars. Even though the masses of these stars differ from each other by no more than 20 per cent, the most massive one increased its luminosity by a factor of about 1000, whereas the smallest one has actually not yet left the main sequence.

It is seen from Fig. 5-16 that less massive stars, smaller than the Sun, will evolve very slowly. Consequently, we shall not consider the evolution

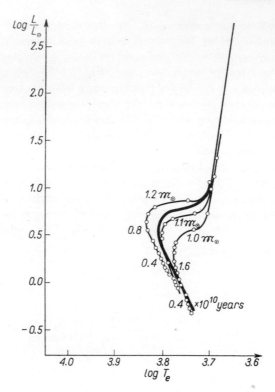

Figure 5-16. Evolutionary tracks and time line [After I. Iben, and J. Faulkner, *Astrophys. Journ.* **153**, 104 (1968)].

of these stars, since even the oldest of them—population-II red dwarfs which fill the lower part of the main sequence—are still in the phase of burning hydrogen in the core.

As soon as a star reaches its maximum brightness, reactions converting helium to heavier elements begin in its core. Further evolution, after a helium core containing the bulk of the stellar mass is formed, proceeds along a horizontal branch of the H–R diagram (with brightness remaining more or less constant, the effective temperature of the star changes). In this phase, energy is produced mainly by helium reactions, while any contribution from the "hydrogen-burning" layer surrounding the core steadily decreases in importance. As it traverses the horizontal branch, the star becomes an RR Lyrae variable for a while.

At the time of writing, the further evolution of the star had not yet been investigated thoroughly, mainly owing to difficulties encountered in building appropriate models of its interior.

Section 54   The Final Evolutionary Phase—The White Dwarf
or the Neutron Star

When the sources of thermonuclear energy have been exhausted, the star becomes less bright and rapidly moves down the H–R diagram to the region occupied by white dwarfs.

The degenerate core previously formed now comprises almost the entire star. It is surrounded by a thin nondegenerate envelope which in general has a thickness of no more than 1 per cent of the stellar radius. As in the case of a star composed of an ideal gas, we can calculate a model of the white dwarf, except that now we use the equation of state for a degenerate gas. In particular, we can find the radius and central density of a white dwarf as a function of its mass. The results of such calculations are listed in Table 5-3.

TABLE 5-3

Relation Between Mass, Radius and Central Density of
White Dwarf

$\mathfrak{M}/\mathfrak{M}_\odot$	$R/R_\odot$	ρ_c (g/cm^3)
0.22	2.0×10^{-2}	2.5×10^5
0.40	1.5×10^{-2}	1.1×10^6
0.50	1.4×10^{-2}	2.0×10^6
0.61	1.2×10^{-2}	3.6×10^6
0.74	1.1×10^{-2}	7.1×10^6
0.88	9.3×10^{-3}	1.6×10^7
1.08	7.1×10^{-3}	5.2×10^7
1.22	5.5×10^{-3}	1.6×10^8
1.33	3.9×10^{-3}	6.8×10^8
1.38	3.0×10^{-3}	2.0×10^9
1.44	0	∞

(After Chandrasekhar, *Stellar Structure*, University of Chicago Press, Chicago, Ill, 1938).

It is seen from this table that the mass of a white dwarf must be less than $1.44 \mathfrak{M}_\odot$. A sphere of greater mass, composed of degenerate gas, would be unstable and hence could not exist. Thus, we can conclude that more massive stars must eject part of their mass at some stage in their evolution, before reaching the white dwarf stage.

The more massive white dwarf stars have smaller radii (Cf. Table 5-3). This is the result of stronger gravitational influences in more massive stars. The amount of energy a star radiates in a unit of time depends on its effective temperature and its surface (hence, on its radius). Thus, on the H–R diagram, more massive white dwarfs will occupy positions below those of less massive ones. The situation is illustrated by Fig. 5-17.

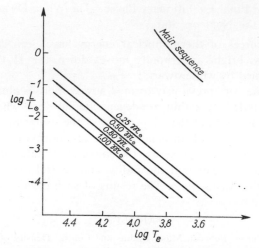

Figure 5-17. A theoretical H–R diagram for white dwarfs [After Martin Schwarzschild, *Structure and Evolution of the Stars* (copyright (c) 1958 by Princeton University Press); reprinted by permission of Princeton University Press].

As time passes, the white dwarfs cool and their temperature and brightness decrease. They move along lines of identical mass from left to right in Fig. 5-17. Table 5-4 lists the luminosity and temperature of a white dwarf of solar mass as a function of the time τ which has elapsed since nuclear reactions ceased in it.

TABLE 5-4

Luminosity and Temperature as a Function of the Cooling Time of a White Dwarf

$L/L_{\odot}$	T (°K)	τ (years)
10^{-2}	17×10^6	0.3×10^9
10^{-3}	9×10^6	1.6×10^9
10^{-4}	4×10^6	8×10^9

(After Martin Schwarzschild, *Structure and Evolution of the Stars* (copyright (c) 1958 by Princeton University Press); reprinted by permission of Princeton University Press).

In the first 1.6×10^9 years after nuclear reactions have stopped, the magnitude of the white dwarf falls off by more than 2^m5. Its brightness will continue to decrease, so that at a certain moment it becomes unobservable. There is another probable end to a star's evolution. In this alternative, the star would go through a supernova state in the final stages of its evolution; after the supernova explosion and ejection of the outermost parts, the core would collapse into a neutron star, a pulsar. This evolutionary track may perhaps be followed by more massive stars, having initial masses several times that of the Sun.

These are the last known stages of changes undergone by matter in the Galaxy. Initially in a dispersed form, this matter—after the formation of stars—passes through the entire cycle of evolution to the state in which it is stored in the cores of white dwarfs and neutron stars.

Section 55   The Influence of Stellar Evolution on Interstellar Matter

We stated earlier that in the course of their evolution, stars eject part of their mass. This is the cause of continuous change in the chemical composition of interstellar matter. The portions of gas ejected by stars are richer in helium and metals than is the matter from which stars were formed. It may be expected that in the period immediately after formation of the Galaxy, when stars began to come into being, interstellar matter contained a much higher percentage of hydrogen than it does at present. The chemical composition of the primeval diffuse matter should be approximately the same as in the atmospheres of the oldest population-II stars. The atmospheres of younger stars, on the other hand, have a chemical composition similar to that which interstellar matter has at present. Hence, we may conclude that at the time when population-II stars were being formed, the abundance of heavy elements in interstellar matter was insignificant.

When discussing Fig. 5-6, we stated that clusters M 3 and M 67, which probably do not differ much in age, belong to different populations. This

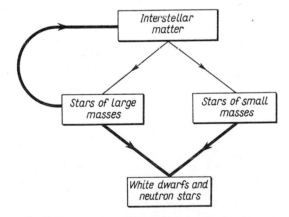

Figure 5-18. Rotation of matter in the Galaxy. → the path of matter with low content of heavy elements, → the path of matter with a high content of heavy elements.

is an argument supporting the view that the process of interstellar matter becoming richer in heavy elements must have been rapid. Population-II stars must have been formed in a relatively short time; evolving rapidly, the more massive of these ejected a considerable fraction of their mass, enriched in metals during nuclear reactions occurring in these stars. Population-I stars then formed out of the interstellar matter which was now more abundant in metals. The cycle of transformations which matter in the Galaxy undergoes can be depicted schematically as in Fig. 5-18.

At the same time as this enrichment in heavy elements was taking place, the amount of diffused interstellar matter probably decreased. This would be so because only part of the matter comprising stars is returned to the interstellar medium; the rest is stored in the interiors of white dwarfs and neutron stars.

THE DISTRIBUTION AND MOTION OF STARS IN THE GALAXY

Section 56   Subsystems of Stars

Studies of the motion of various types of stars in space, on the basis of measurements of radial velocities and proper motions, have made it possible to establish a relationship between the kinetic properties and physical features of stars. By way of illustration, Fig. 5-19 shows the relation between the mean radial velocity with respect to the Sun and the spectral type of the star. The solid line represents main-sequence stars, the dashed line, giants.

The difference which can be seen on Fig. 5-19 between the velocities of stars of various spectral types and the particularly distinct separation of red giants and supergiants from the red dwarfs which belong to the main

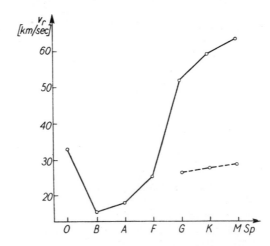

Figure 5-19. Mean radial velocities vs. spectral types of stars.

sequence are indicative that classification of stars into groups according to their kinematical features is possible and that this corresponds approximately to our previous classification of stars according to their physical properties. For this reason, a test based on a study of the motion of stars and their distribution in space may prove very useful when effecting a population classification.

Of course, the mean radial velocity presented in Fig. 5-19 is not the only feature which should be taken into account in such considerations. Classification may be based on any feature or group of independent kinematical features which sufficiently differentiate the congregation of all stars in the Galaxy into groups of stars related to each other by common physical properties, evolution, etc.

If, for instance, we were to draw the velocity vectors of two groups of stars lying near the Sun—one group belonging to population-I and the other to population-II—we would get diagrams as in Figs. 5-20 and 5-21. It is seen from Fig. 5-20 that the population-I stars have low ve-

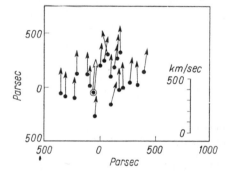

Figure 5-20. Velocities of population-I stars.

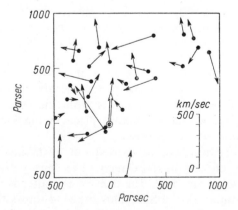

Figure 5-21. Velocities of population-II stars.

locities relative to the Sun and, hence, the dispersion of their velocities is not great. Population-II stars, on the other hand, display a considerable dispersion of velocities, in regard to both absolute value and direction.

A measure of the dispersion of the velocities $\mathbf{v}_i$ of a group of n stars may be given by the expression

$$\sigma = \sqrt{\frac{\sum_{i=1}^{n} (\mathbf{v}_i - \mathbf{v}_0)^2}{n}}, \qquad (5\text{-}34)$$

where $\mathbf{v}_0$, the mean velocity of stars belonging to that group, is

$$\mathbf{v}_0 = \frac{\sum_{i=1}^{n} \mathbf{v}_i}{n}. \qquad (5\text{-}35)$$

Table 5-5 lists the mean abundance Z of metals and the velocity dispersion σ for several groups of stars.

TABLE 5-5

Abundance of Metals and Velocity Dispersion for
Several Groups of Stars

Objects	Z	σ (km/sec)
Young galactic clusters	0.04	10
Stars with strong metallic lines	0.03	20
Stars with weak metallic lines	0.02	30
High-velocity stars	0.01	50
Globular clusters	0.003	130

(On basis of Schwarzschild, *Stellar Populations*, Ed. by O'Connell, Vatican Observatory, 207, 1958).

We thus see that the velocity spread σ of a given group of stars may be used as a criterion for classification. On the other hand, the fact that the velocity spread decreases as we pass from the oldest objects to the youngest is evidence of changes taking place in the kinematics of the Galaxy in the course of its evolution.

A similar classification can be carried out by taking the distribution of particular types of stars in the Galaxy. The density distribution in the Galaxy is presented in Fig. 5-22. The density of matter is taken arbitrarily as one in the proximity of the Sun. This drawing shows the cross-section of the Galaxy in the direction perpendicular to the plane of maximum

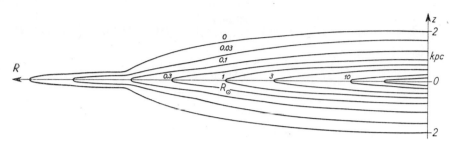

Figure 5-22. Schematic distribution of density in the Galaxy. $R_\odot$—position of the Sun. The numbers denote the relative density of matter in relation to the density in the vicinity of the Sun [After Schmidt, *Bull. Astron. Inst. Netherlands XIII*, 15 (1956)].

density, the plane of the galactic equator. The Galaxy plane is the principal plane in the galactic system of astronomical coordinates. The principal direction in this system is the direction towards the centre of the Galaxy, the site of maximum density in the Galaxy. The angle U (Cf. Sec. 5) is called the galactic longitude, while the angle V is known as the galactic latitude.

A density distribution diagram drawn in a similar fashion for a chosen group of stars would be different in appearance. Groups of stars selected according to physical features constitute systems which, to a lesser or greater extent, concentrate about the plane of the Galaxy. A measure of the concentration of stars about the galactic plane may be given by the expression

$$\left| \frac{\partial \log \mathscr{D}}{\partial z} \right|, \tag{5-36}$$

where $\mathscr{D}$ is the density of stars of the type under consideration*, and z is the distance from the Galaxy plane. In regard to the value of expression (5-36), we classify stars as those belonging to flat subsystems $\left(\text{large} \left| \frac{\partial \log \mathscr{D}}{\partial z} \right| \right)$, intermediate, or spherical subsystems $\left(\text{small} \left| \frac{\partial \log \mathscr{D}}{\partial z} \right| \right)$. An ancillary criterion in a classification of this kind may be given by the value of the expression

$$\left| \frac{\partial \log \mathscr{D}}{\partial R} \right| \tag{5-37}$$

where R is the projection of the distance from the Galaxy centre onto the Galaxy plane.

* This is the number of stars of a given type per unit volume.

The values of $\left|\dfrac{\partial \log \mathscr{D}}{z}\right|$ and $\left|\dfrac{\partial \log \mathscr{D}}{R}\right|$ for several groups of objects are given in Table 5-6.

TABLE 5-6

Subsystems of Stars

Subsystem	$\left\|\dfrac{\partial \log \mathscr{D}}{\partial z}\right\|$	$\left\|\dfrac{\partial \log \mathscr{D}}{\partial R}\right\|$
Flat subsystems:		
Type-O stars	7.5	0.10
Open clusters	8.2	0.11
Long-period cepheids	9.9	0.11
Intermediate subsystems:		
Planetary nebulae	2.0	0.4
Long-period variables	0.9	0.26
Spherical subsystems:		
Short-period cepheids	0.22	0.27
Globular clusters	0.15	0.26

(On basis of Zonn and Rudnicki, *Astronomia Gwiaz-dowa* (Stellar Astronomy), PWN—Polish Scientific Publishers, Warsaw, 1957).

All objects belonging to flat subsystems are population-I objects, while all objects of spherical subsystems belong to population-II.

The division into populations by kinematical criteria, is of course, not as good as classification using the physical features of the individual stars. This is so because the former does not permit the population membership of individual objects to be determined, but merely may be applied statistically to groups of stars previously separated on the basis of morphological features. On the other hand, it does have the advantage that it is not as labour-consuming and can be performed quickly for a large number of stars.

The finding that old stars (population-II) comprise a spherical subsystem, while young stars (population-I) are concentrated about the galactic plane (which at present contains the bulk of interstellar matter) indicates that stars were initially also formed far from the galactic plane. This would mean that regions occupied by interstellar gas were at one time extended much further than at present, and that as population-II was formed, the interstellar matter was concentrated increasingly in a narrow layer where star-forming processes are still taking place. Present data do not yet make it possible to determine what thermal and dynamic conditions prevailed in the gas which originally constituted the Galaxy, nor how the Galaxy evolved to the present state.

Section 57   Galactic Rotation

In the preceding section we found that the motion of various groups of stars with respect to the Sun is not the same. In particular, population-II objects are characterized by high velocities relative to the Sun and a large velocity dispersion, whereas the velocities of objects of the extreme population I do not in general exceed twenty km/sec. Let us consider this is greater detail.

A mean velocity v_0 relative to the Sun can be calculated from Eq. (5-35) for every group of stars, selected according to their morphological features. The difference $v_i - v_0$ between the velocity of a star and the mean velocity of the group is called the peculiar velocity of the star (Cf. Fig. 5-23).

Mean velocities are plotted in Fig. 5-24 for a number of groups of

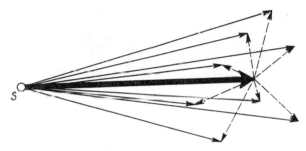

Figure 5-23. The mean velocity of groups of stars →, peculiar velocities ⇢, the velocities of stars relative to the Sun →.

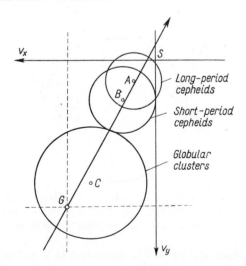

Figure 5-24. Strömberg diagram [On the basis of Strömberg, *Astrophys Journ.* **61**, 353 (1925)].

stars from the immediate neighbourhood of the Sun. A diagram so drawn is called a Strömberg diagram. In its construction, only stellar velocity components parallel to the galactic plane were taken into account. The centres of circles in Fig. 5-24 correspond to the mean velocities of the given star groups with respect to the Sun. The radii of these circles are equal to the magnitude of the dispersion of the peculiar velocities possessed by the stars in each group. The Strömberg diagram shows that even though individual star groups move in space with different velocities, there never-theless is a certain pivileged direction for their motion (marked by an arrow in the drawing).

If stars moved through space in straight lines (or, in general, on un-bounded curves), a state would soon be reached such that groups of stars moving at different velocities would become separated (Fig. 5-25). A Gal-

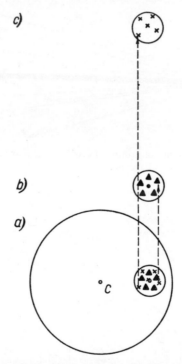

Figure 5-25. The hypothesis of rectilinear motions of stars: a) the present appearance of the Galaxy; b) the future position of stars moving with low velocities; c) the future position of stars mowing with high velocities.

axy such as we observe now would thus—if the hypothesis of rectilinear motion of the stars were accepted—be an eminently unstable object, a chance meeting place of various types of stars. Moreover, there would be no reason why some privileged direction should exist for the motion of these objects, though this is clearly evident on the Strömberg diagram. A Galaxy lifetime as short as would emerge from the assumption of rectilinear motions by the stars (of the order of 10^8 years) is in contradiction with the conclusions drawn about the age of the Galaxy from the theory of stellar evolution and incompatible with the regularity of the Galactic structure. For these reasons, we must reject the hypothesis that the stars move in straight lines.

All of these difficulties involved in interpreting the Strömberg diagram disappear when we accept the hypothesis of galactic rotation (Fig. 5-26).

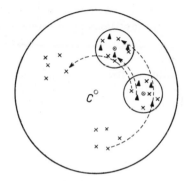

Figure 5-26. Stars circling about the nucleus of the Galaxy at different velocities.

The direction marked on the Strömberg diagram by an arrow shows the direction of stellar revolution in the Galaxy, perpendicular to the direction towards the galactic centre. The revolution of stars about the galactic centre proves the existence of forces which impart to the stars accelerations causing them to change direction in their motion, thus, indirectly this confirms the applicability of the law of universal gravitation to bodies thousands of parsecs apart.

The origin of the coordinate system in Fig. 5-24 corresponds to zero stellar velocity with respect to the Sun. However, the Sun also participates in the rotation of the Galaxy and it would be more correct to measure the velocities of the stars with respect to some fictitious point not involved in the galactic rotation. The position of such a point could be determined from the velocities of objects which do not belong to our Galaxy, e.g. from the observed velocities of other galaxies. If we were to assume that our Galaxy does not have any systematic motion with respect to all the galaxies as a whole, the origin of the coordinate system in Fig. 5-24 would have to be moved to a point corresponding to the mean velocity of the galaxies with respect to the Sun (the coordinate system fixed at this point is indicated by dashed lines in Fig. 5-24). We then find that the stars of flat subsystems revolve around the galactic centre with the highest velocities, while the velocity of rotation of spherical subsystems is low.

The differences in the velocities of rotation of different subsystems stem from the fact that stars in flat subsystems move in nearly circular orbits which lie almost exactly in the plane of the Galaxy, while stars belonging to spherical subsystems move in eccentric orbits which are inclined to the galactic plane and have a large dispersion of eccentricities and inclination angles. Consequently, whereas groups of stars belonging to flat subsystems have mean velocities of revolution around the galactic centre which are almost equal to the velocities of the individual stars, the value of the mean resultant velocity of spherical subsystems is much smaller than the absolute value of the velocities of the individual member objects.

The velocity of rotation in the Galaxy (the magnitude of the angular velocity) changes with distance from the centre (differential rotation). These changes can be analysed more exactly on the basis of observations of stellar motion in various directions around the Sun.

By virtue of Fig. 5-27 we can write the relations

$$R\sin(l+\alpha) = R_\odot\sin l, \tag{5-38}$$

$$\left.\begin{aligned} v_r &= \omega(R)\,R\sin(l+\alpha) \\ v_{r\odot} &= \omega(R_\odot)\,R_\odot\sin l \end{aligned}\right\}, \tag{5-39}$$

where $R_\odot$ and R, respectively, denote the distance of the Sun and the star (lying in the galactic plane) from the centre of the Galaxy, α is the

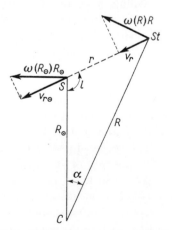

Figure 5-27. A sketch for determining Oort's constant. S—Sun, St—star, C—centre of the Galaxy.

angle between the radius vectors of the Sun and the star, and l is the galactic longitude of the star (the angle between the directions to the galactic centre and to the given star). Assuming that the given star and the Sun move in circles around the centre of the Galaxy (and bearing in mind that the relative radial velocity Δv_r is negative when the star approaches the Sun), we can calculate the relative radial velocity Δv_r by using Eqs. (5-38) and (5-39) as follows:

$$\Delta v_r = -(v_r - v_{r\odot}) = -[\omega(R)\,R\sin(l+\alpha) - \omega(R_\odot)\,R_\odot\sin l]$$
$$= -[\omega(R)\,R_\odot\sin l - \omega(R_\odot)\,R_\odot\sin l]$$
$$= -R_\odot[\omega(R) - \omega(R_\odot)]\sin l, \tag{5-40}$$

where $\omega(R)$ is the angular velocity of rotation at a distance R from the centre. If we confine ourselves to considering the motion of stars near the Sun ($r \ll R_\odot$), we can expand the expression in brackets into a Taylor series and consider only terms of the first order

$$\omega(R) - \omega(R_\odot) = \left[\frac{d\omega(R)}{dR}\right]_{R=R_\odot}(R-R_\odot) + \frac{1}{2}\left[\frac{d^2\omega(R)}{dR^2}\right]_{R=R_\odot} \times$$

$$\times (R-R_\odot)^2 + \ldots \approx \left[\frac{d\omega(R)}{dR}\right]_{R=R_\odot}(R-R_\odot). \tag{5-41}$$

Since for small r's we have

$$R - R_\odot \approx -r\cos l \tag{5-42}$$

then formula (5-40) can be rewritten as

$$\Delta v_r \approx R_\odot\left[\frac{d\omega(R)}{dR}\right]_{R=R_\odot}r\cos l\sin l = rA\sin 2l, \tag{5-43}$$

where

$$A = \frac{1}{2}R_\odot\left[\frac{d\omega(R)}{dR}\right]_{R=R_\odot} \tag{5-44}$$

is Oort's constant.

From Eq. (5-43) we find that in the case when there is differential rotation of the Galaxy, the diagram of stellar radial velocities as a function of the galactic longitude should be a double sine curve. Stars lying in the direction of the centre and anticentre, and in directions perpendicular to these directions, should have zero radial velocity, whereas stars observed in directions differing by 45° from those mentioned should have maximum radial velocity. Knowing the distance r of the given group of stars from the Sun, we can measure the amplitude of the sine curve obtained in order to find the constant A which determines the change in the velocity of rotation near the Sun.

Figure 5-28 presents the radial velocity diagrams for four groups of cepheids. The stars of group 1 are, on the average, 420 pc from the Sun, of group 2—1060 pc, group 3—1660 pc, and group 4—2310 pc. We can use Fig. 5-28 to determine the value of the constant A. This value, obtained

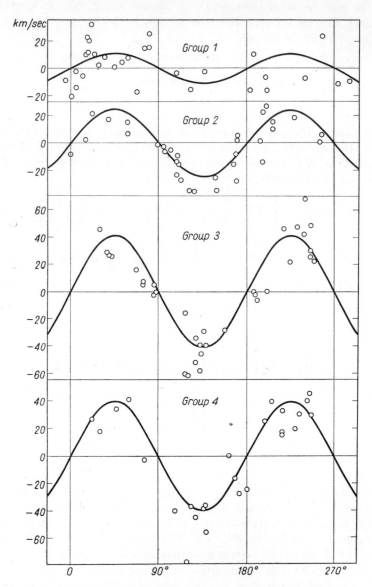

Figure 5-28. Observed radial velocities as a function of the galactic long.
itude [On the basis of Joy, *Astrophys. Journ.* **89**, 356 (1939)].

on the basis of present-day measurements, is $+15$ km/sec · kpc. The fact that $A > 0$ means that $\left[\dfrac{d\omega(R)}{dR}\right]_{R=R_\odot} > 0$. However, since the absolute value of the angular velocity may not increase as a function of R, therefore $\omega(R_\odot) < 0$, which signifies that the Galaxy rotates in a clockwise direction in a system of coordinates such as adopted in Fig. 5-27.

Let us return to Eq. (5-40). The expression

$$f(R, R_\odot) = R_\odot[\omega(R) - \omega(R_\odot)] \tag{5-45}$$

is known as the Camm function. The values of this function can be calculated from the formula

$$f(R, R_\odot) = \Delta v_r \cosec l \tag{5-46}$$

if we know the radial velocities of stars at various distances from the galactic centre. In determining the values of the Camm function, we must confine ourselves to the radial velocities of stars which move in, or close to, the galactic plane inasmuch, as we know, the stars of spherical subsystems have a different, smaller, velocity of rotation. On the other hand, corrections must be made to the radial velocities because the Sun and the observed stars do not move exactly in circles.

Knowledge of the Camm function enables us to determine the rotational velocity from Eq. (5-45) as a function of the distance from the galactic centre.

Considerable advances have been made in investigations on the rotation of the Galaxy since long-distance radio observations of interstellar gas first began. The motion of interstellar gas, a typical component of a flat subsystem, is a particularly good example of circular motion in the galactic plane.

The principle involved in finding the rotational velocity from radio observations of interstellar hydrogen is as follows. Measurements give us the magnitude of the Doppler shift of the 21-cm line* observed from various directions in the Galaxy (Sec. 64). From this we calculate the maximum radial velocity of the gas with respect to the Sun as a function of the galactic longitude. If the gas is assumed to move in circles around the nucleus of the Galaxy, then a ring of matter moving about the galactic centre in a circle tangent to the line of sight (Cf. Fig. 5-29) has maximum radial velocity.

Since

$$R = R_\odot \sin l \tag{5-47}$$

---

* Radiation in this line is produced when the direction of the electron spin is reversed with respect to the spin of the nucleus (proton) in the hydrogen atom.

then when we use Eq. (5-47) to find the distance from the galactic centre to that ring of maximum radial velocity with respect to the Sun, we can find ω from Eq. (5-40). Repeating this procedure for all values of l, we obtain $\omega(R)$, the distribution of the rotational velocity as a function of the distance from the centre of the Galaxy. Figure 5-30 presents an angular velocity diagram found in this way, while Fig. 5-31 shows the diagram of the linear velocity of galactic rotation.

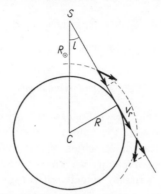

Figure 5-29. Diagram of the circular motion of gas in the Galaxy.

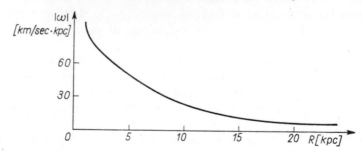

Figure 5-30. Angular velocity vs. distance from the centre of the Galaxy.

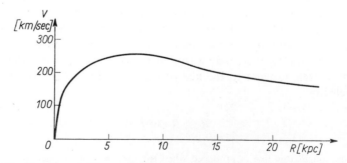

Figure 5-31. Circular velocity vs. distance from the centre of the Galaxy.

Section 58   Mass Distribution in the Galaxy

The kinetic theory of galactic rotation presented in the preceding section provides a basis for determining the gravitational potential and, indirectly, the distribution of mass in the Galaxy. The density distribution in the Galaxy was delineated in Fig. 5-22. Characteristic features of the density distribution in the Galaxy as shown in that drawing were the existence of a massive nucleus located at the centre of a very flat disk of radius exceeding 16 kpc and a thickness of merely $\frac{1}{2}$ kpc or thereabouts. The Sun is about 10 kpc from the centre, and lies almost exactly in the plane of the Galaxy. The total mass of the Galaxy is of the order of 10^{11} solar masses, or of the order of 10^{44} g.

The distribution of young objects inside the galactic disk reveals a tendency on their part to form concentrations which could be identified with the spiral arms of the Galaxy. The position of the observed associations is illustrated in Fig. 5-32; the shape of the spiral arms can be seen.

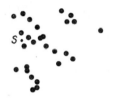

Figure 5-32. Distribution of associations in the vicinity of the Sun. *S*—Sun; *C*—centre of the Galaxy.

The spiral structure of the Galaxy is much more distinctly evident in the distribution of hydrogen in the Galaxy. This is a subject which will be discussed in our next chapter. The fact that a spiral structure can be distinguished in the distribution of young objects and that the position of the spiral arms formed by these objects coincides with the gaseous spiral arms constitutes one more premise testifying to the genetic relation between interstellar matter and young stars.

Chapter 6   Interstellar Matter

In the preceding chapter, we pointed out the important role interstellar matter plays in the evolution of the Galaxy. Since stars form out of this matter, its state, distribution and motion in the Galaxy exert a decisive influence on the kinematics of stellar subsystems which come into being and on the structure of young stars (chemical composition) belonging to those subsystems. This is undoubtedly why in recent years astronomers have been showing a steadily growing interest in interstellar matter. Investigations into interstellar matter have been intensified considerably, thanks to the radio observations which began after World War II. These observations make it possible to reach out to extremely distant regions and provide a basis for determining the distribution of interstellar gas in the Galaxy. Optical observations provided information about the physical conditions, the chemical composition, and the properties of the interstellar matter in the neighbourhood of the Sun.

Section 59   Evidence of Interstellar Matter

The observational methods of confirming the presence of matter diffused throughout interstellar space are as follows:

1. The existence of bright nebulae which can be seen on photographs of the sky.

2. The occurrence of dark clouds.

3. The failure to observe galaxies in the vicinity of the plane of the Milky Way.

4. The increasing reddening of starlight with distance.

5. The presence of lines of interstellar origin in the stellar spectra.

6. Polarization of starlight.

7. Observation of radio emission.

At present, we shall discuss points 1–5, leaving the discussion of points 6 and 7 to later sections in this chapter.

1. The Orion nebula shown in Plate 23 is an example of a luminous gas cloud.

2. In the middle of the segment of the sky shown in Plate 24 is a region in which only a few stars can be seen. This is due to the existence of a dense cloud of interstellar matter which obscures the stars lying beyond it. In adjoining regions not obscured by interstellar matter, we see remote stars

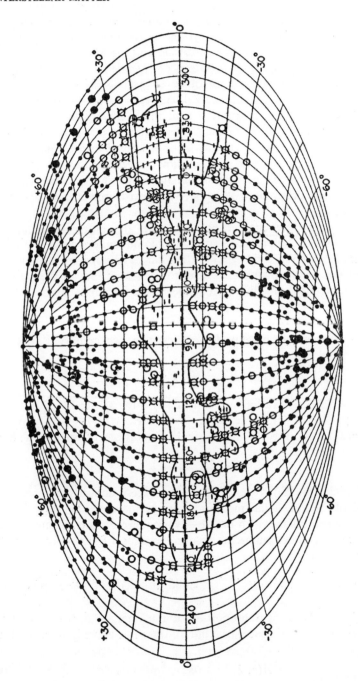

Figure 6-1. Hubble's illustration of the zone of avoidance.

and the density of stars observed in the photograph is high. Several stars which can be seen against the background of the cloud are stars which lie on this side of the cloud, between the cloud and the Sun.

3. Much data about the distribution of interstellar matter can be obtained by counting the number of observed galaxies as a function of the galactic longitude. The number of galaxies seen in a field of one square degree of arc is found to be greatest near the galactic poles, decreasing as we approach the plane of the Galaxy. No galaxies at all are observed below $10°$ galactic lattitude (Fig. 6-1). This zone is known as the zone of avoidance. Since the distribution of galaxies cannot be related to the orientation of our Galaxy in space, the only explanation for what we observe is that matter which obscures objects lying beyond it exists in a narrow layer about the galactic plane.

4. In the preceding chapter, we spoke of the difference in absolute magnitudes in two colours of some star (colour index) being a function of the temperature (spectral type) of that star. The apparent magnitude of a star depends on the distance r from the observer and on the extinction $A(r)$ of the interstellar medium, according to the formula

$$m = M - 5 + 5\log r + A(r). \tag{6-1}$$

Thus, the difference in magnitudes observed in two colours λ_1 and λ_2 is given by the relation

$$m(\lambda_1) - m(\lambda_2) = M(\lambda_1) - M(\lambda_2) + A(r, \lambda_1) - A(r, \lambda_2). \tag{6-2}$$

By spectroscopic observations we can establish the spectral type of the star and thus indirectly determine the colour index $M(\lambda_1) - M(\lambda_2)$. We find $m(\lambda_1) - m(\lambda_2)$ from direct photometrical observations of brightness; hence, the colour excess

$$A(r, \lambda_1) - A(r, \lambda_2) \tag{6-3}$$

can be found from Eq. (6-2). The colour excess depends on the optical properties of the interstellar medium or, to be more precise, on the optical thickness for colours in which the observations were made. Using Eq. (5-9) from Ch. 5, we can determine the colour excess as a function of the optical thickness. Namely,

$$A(r, \lambda) = -2.5 \log e^{-\tau_\lambda(r)} = 1.085\tau_\lambda(r) = 1.085 \int_0^r \varkappa_\lambda \varrho(r)\,dr. \tag{6-4}$$

Assuming that the optical properties of the interstellar material are the same throughout all of space, i.e. that $\varkappa_\lambda$ does not depend on r, we obtain

$$A(r, \lambda) = 1.085\varkappa_\lambda \int_0^r \varrho(r)\,dr. \tag{6-5}$$

Thus, inserting Eq. (6-5) into the expression (6-3), we have

$$A(r, \lambda_1) - A(r, \lambda_2) = 1.085[\varkappa(\lambda_1) - \varkappa(\lambda_2)] \int_0^r \varrho(r) dr. \qquad (6\text{-}6)$$

When we divide Eq. (6-6) by Eq. (6-5), we arrive at

$$\frac{A(r, \lambda_1) - A(r, \lambda_2)}{A(r, \lambda)} = \frac{\varkappa(\lambda_1) - \varkappa(\lambda_2)}{\varkappa(\lambda)} = f(\lambda_1, \lambda_2, \lambda). \qquad (6\text{-}7)$$

We see that this ratio does not depend on the density of the interstellar medium, nor on the path traversed by the light ray, but only on the set of colours in which the observations were made. For each photometric system, that is, for fixed λ_1, λ_2, and λ, the right-hand side of Eq. (6-7) is constant and, hence the colour excess increases with distance in proportion to the extinction. For the nearer stars, whose distances have been calculated by methods not requiring knowledge of extinction, we can determine the colour excess and extinction independently, and thus find the value of the function $f(\lambda_1, \lambda_2, \lambda)$ for the photometric system employed. Using this value for all stars, including those whose distance from the Sun is not known, we can find the interstellar extinction from Eq. (6-7) after measuring the colour excess and then find the distance to the star from Eq. (6-1).

Important information about the interstellar medium can be obtained by studying the dependence of interstellar extinction on the wavelength of the light (Fig. 6-2). We see that for radiation with a wavelength of 0.3 μ

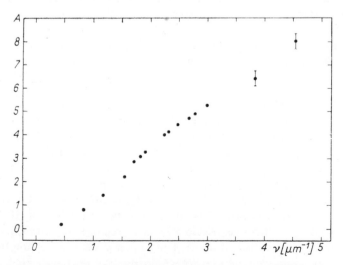

Figure 6-2. Dependence of interstellar extinction on the wavelength of light [On the basis of Bogges and Borgman, *Astrophys. Journ.* **140**, 1636 (1964)].

to 1 μ extinction is almost exactly proportion to λ^{-1}. We can thus draw conclusions from this about the size of the particles responsible for interstellar extinction. If the extinction were caused by particles 10^{-6} cm or smaller in size, then according to Rayleigh's scattering law, $\varkappa(\lambda)$ would have to be proportional to λ^{-4}. Particles with a size of 10^{-4} cm or more would cause nonselective scattering (independent of the wavelength). Only in the case of particles measuring 10^{-5} cm is the scattering proportional to λ^{-1}, which is in agreement with observation. We may thus conclude that one of the components of interstellar matter is dust with grains of the order of 10^{-5} cm. Starlight passing through such a dust medium is scattered more strongly for shorter waves—blue light, and less for longer waves—red light. For this reason, a star observed through a dust cloud appears redder than it is in actual fact. This is why this phenomenon is called interstellar reddening.

5. The spectra of many stars are observed to contain absorption lines which we have reason to suppose were not produced in the stellar atmospheres. This is indicated by the fact that the Doppler shift of these lines differs from that of the stellar lines. Thus, the gas in which they came into being must have been moving with a different velocity with respect to the observer than was the star. Such lines observed in the spectra of pulsating stars, unlike the lines produced in the photospheres, do not alter their position in rhythm with variations in the stellar brightness. These lines are narrower than the stellar lines, which indicates that they were produced in a more rarefied medium with a lower temperature.

Plate 25 shows the spectra of some stars with interstellar lines. Note that each of these spectra has lines which are split into two or three components. This testifies to the fact that the light passed through a medium in which absorption occurred in two or three clouds moving at different velocities.

Section 60   Interstellar Clouds

The remarks made in the preceding Section lead us to the conclusion that interstellar matter is not a homogeneous medium but occurs in the form of a number of condensations—clouds, which must collide with each other as they move through space. Such collisions will be accompanied by the disintegration of the clouds, and the escape of matter from them into the surrounding medium. The mean lifetime of one cloud (i.e. the time between two successive collisions) may be estimated at 10^7 years from knowledge of the size of clouds, their relative velocities, and the number of clouds per unit volume. Thus, if new ones were not formed, the number of clouds in the Galaxy would quickly decrease. Hence, processes in which new clouds are formed and old ones disintegrated must be taking place continuously, and during these processes gas moves from the intercloud regions into the clouds and is once again scattered in space.

If a bright hot star happens to be near or inside a cloud the radiation of this star will be capable of exciting the atoms of the gas constituting the cloud so that they glow. The cloud will then be observed as a bright nebula possessing a typical gas spectrum consisting of separate emission lines characteristic of the gas comprising the cloud. It is a different matter if the illuminating star is cool. In that case the atoms of the gas will not be excited and the gas will not glow but the cloud is visible because of radiation scattered on grains of dust. The spectrum of light from this nebula is a reflection of the spectrum of the illuminating star. Dark nebulae are ones which have no illuminating star nearby. They can be detected only when they occur against the background of starry regions of the Milky Way or from reddening of light or the presence of absorption lines in the spectra of stars situated beyond them.

It is seen, therefore, that the appearance of a nebula, its luminosity and spectrum, depend on the chance meeting of a star and a cloud of gas and dust. There is no genetic relation between an illuminating star and the cloud it illuminates. However, it is known from evolutionary theory that stars (at least, the more massive ones) lost part of their mass at a certain stage in their life. We should accordingly expect there to be stars which are surrounded by clouds of gas formed by their recently ejected outer parts. And indeed, such nebulae do exist and are known as planetary nebulae (Plate 26). Analysis of the Doppler shifts of the spectral lines of planetary nebula reveals that the nebula surrounding the star is expanding. This is an argument in favour of the existence of a genetic relation between the cloud and the star.

Section 61   Ionization

As stated above, hot stars are capable of exciting nearby gas to luminescence. This takes place as a result of gas atoms being bombarded with high-energy photons whose energy is higher than the ionization energy of the gas atoms. Hydrogen, the main constituent of interstellar matter, has an ionization potential of 13.6 ev. This is the energy carried by quanta of radiation with a wavelength of

$$\lambda = hc/E = 912 \text{ Å}. \tag{6-8}$$

Radiation of a wavelength shorter than 912 Å ionizes hydrogen atoms. The free electrons released in this way recombine with hydrogen nuclei (protons) and, occupying one of the levels, emit their excess energy. As they fall to lower and lower energy levels they produce a whole series of hydrogen lines. Thus, at any time, some of the atoms will be ionized, and some will be neutral (un-ionized). What fraction of all atoms is ionized depends on the ionization and recombination rates. Ionization equilibrium is established in the medium when the recombination rate is equal to the ionization rate.

The ionization rate $\mathscr{I}$ is proportional to the number of quanta of ionizing radiation (with $\lambda < 912$ Å) and the density of neutral hydrogen atoms

$$\mathscr{I} = A n_{\mathrm{H}} \mathscr{E}, \tag{6-9}$$

where A is a constant of proportionality.

The recombination rate $\mathscr{R}$ is proportional to the density n_e of electrons and n_p of protons

$$\mathscr{R} = B n_e n_p, \tag{6-10}$$

where B is a constant of proportionality.

If by x we denote the degree of ionization (the ratio of ionized atoms to the total number of atoms)

$$x = \frac{n_p}{n} = \frac{n_p}{n_{\mathrm{H}} + n_p}, \tag{6-11}$$

and if we assume that the gas is electrically neutral,

$$n_p = n_e, \tag{6-12}$$

then the condition for ionization equilibrium

$$\mathscr{R} = \mathscr{I} \tag{6-13}$$

can be written as

$$B n^2 x^2 = A(1-x) n \mathscr{E}. \tag{6-14}$$

The illumination $\mathscr{E}$ at a given point can be calculated if we know the value $\mathscr{E}_0$ at the surface of the star,

$$\mathscr{E} = \mathscr{E}_0 \left(\frac{R_0}{r} \right)^2 e^{-\tau}, \tag{6-15}$$

where R_0 is the radius of the star, r is the distance from the star to the point under consideration, and τ is the optical thickness of the medium. Since absorption occurs only in the un-ionized hydrogen, therefore

$$\tau = \int_0^r \varkappa n_{\mathrm{H}} m_{\mathrm{H}} \, dr = \int_0^r \varkappa (1-x) n m_{\mathrm{H}} \, dr. \tag{6-16}$$

Thus, inserting Eqs. (6-15) and (6-16) into Eq. (6-14), we obtain

$$x^2 n = C(1-x) r^{-2} e^{-\int_0^r \varkappa (1-x) n m_{\mathrm{H}} dr}, \tag{6-17}$$

where

$$C = \frac{A}{B} R_0^2 \mathscr{E}_0 \tag{6-18}$$

depends on the spectral type, brightness, and radius of the illuminating star.

The gas near the star is ionized almost completely ($x \approx 1$), and consequently the opacity is practically zero in this region. The illumination then decreases as r^{-2} up to a distance when it is too small to cause total ionization of the hydrogen. Opacity increases sharply in the partially ionized medium and the illumination by the ionizing radiation quickly diminishes to zero as $e^{-\tau}$. Apart from a thin region of partial ionization, the rest of the gas will remain neutral. This is illustrated in Fig. 6-3 where the solution of Eq. (6-17) is plotted.

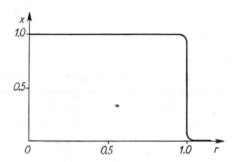

Figure 6-3. Degree of ionization of interstellar hydrogen vs. distance to the illuminating star. The distance is given in radii of the ionized region.

The table below gives the radii of spheres of complete radiation which are formed in a homogeneous hydrogen medium, with a density of 1 atom per cm³, as a function of the spectral type of the ionizing stars.

From the data listed in Table 6-1 we see that spheres of ionized hydrogen form for the most part only around type-*O* stars and stars of the first

TABLE 6-1

Radii of Ionized Regions

Spectral Type of Illuminating Star	Radius (pc)
O5	94
O6	85
O7	78
O8	72
O9	63
B0	46
B1	17
B2	12
B3	6.6
B5	3.6

[After Prentice, ter Haar, MN RAS, **146**, 423 (1969)].

subtypes of type *B*. The radii of these spheres, called Strömgren spheres, depend on the spectral type of the star and the density of the interstellar gas in the region under consideration. The Strömgren spheres have smaller radii when the density of the gas is higher. In view of the small size of the transition layer, containing partially ionized hydrogen gas, we can treat the interstellar gas as though it occurs in regions where it is either completely neutral (H I regions) or completely ionized (H II regions). It should be borne in mind, however, that even in regions of neutral hydrogen there are ionized atoms of heavier elements (carbon, silicon) and free electrons whose presence may be vital in many thermal and electromagnetic processes in interstellar space.

Section 62   Temperature

In this section we consider the major processes determining the temperature of the interstellar gas, with which energy is supplied to the gas as well as those processes which lead to a loss of energy by the gas.

As already stated above, clouds of interstellar gas collide with each other. In consequence of these collisions, the kinetic energy of the moving clouds is expended on heating the gas. Another process which raises the temperature of the clouds is the bombardment of the gas atoms by extremely fast cosmic-ray particles. At the same time, the interaction between interstellar gas and the radiation field of the stars plays an important role in heating the gas.

Let us take a closer look at the latter process. The gas atoms are ionized under the influence of stellar radiation. Electrons which are knocked out carry off an energy equal to the difference between the energy of the ionizing quantum and the ionization energy of the given atom. In general this energy is greater than the mean energy of free electrons in the cloud. When the electrons meet, an equalization of their energies ensues: those recently produced by ionization are faster and lose energy, while the others are slower and gain energy; the gas heats up. After a time the electrons with lower velocities recombine with ions into neutral atoms and the cycle is repeated. As a result, we have a continuous influx of fast electrons which are produced in ionization events and a depletion of slow electrons which are lost in the course of recombination.

The gas cools by radiating energy in those parts of the spectrum in which the interstellar medium is optically transparent. Electrons excite atoms and ions with which they collide, while themselves losing energy. The excited atoms emit radiation at their characteristic frequencies. The interstellar medium is practically transparent for long-wavelength radiation emitted by atoms of heavier elements (mainly oxygen), excited to low-lying energy levels. The energy of this radiation is lost irretrievably by the gas.

Let us consider what elements predominate in the process by which interstellar gas is heated and cooled. Since hydrogen is the principal constituent of interstellar matter, these processes may be expected to proceed in a different manner in clouds of neutral hydrogen (H I) than in clouds of ionized hydrogen (H II). Hence we shall carry out the discussion separately for H I and H II regions.

Heating in H II regions is caused when hydrogen atoms are ionized by radiation with a wavelength shorter than 912 Å. The fact that the medium is almost completely ionized means that the time between consecutive ionizations and recombinations of each atom is much longer than the time which the atom spends in the neutral state. The rate of the heating processes $\mathscr{G}$ depends on the intensity of radiation of wavelengths $\lambda < 912$ Å, that is, on the spectral type of the illuminating star and on the gas temperature (strictly speaking, on the difference between the mean velocity of the free electrons and the mean velocity attained by the electrons during ionization of the hydrogen atoms). Oxygen atoms excited to luminescence in forbidden lines are mainly responsible for the cooling. The cooling rate $\mathscr{L}$ depends on the number of collisions of oxygen atoms with free electrons, or on the velocity of the electrons (temperature), and the number of electrons and oxygen atoms per unit volume. The rates of heating and cooling processes in H II regions are plotted in Fig. 6-4 for various types of illuminating stars.

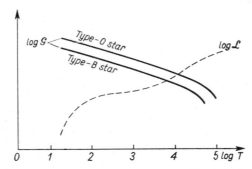

Figure 6-4. The curves of the heating and cooling rates, $\mathscr{G}$ and $\mathscr{L}$, in H II regions.

It is seen from Fig. 6-4 that equilibrium between the heating and cooling rates is established at a gas temperature of about 10,000°K. Hence, this is the temperature H II regions should have.

In H I regions, where neutral hydrogen occurs, heating can take place only by ionization of other elements. The fact that the hydrogen is not ionized indicates that quanta with energies in excess of 13.6 eV do not exist there. Thus, only atoms with a low ionization potential, first and foremost atoms of carbon and silicon, can be ionized. However, since these elements are much less abundant than hydrogen in interstellar matter, the rate of heating processes will be much lower in H I regions and in H II regions. Cooling is effected by excitation of carbon, iron, and sulphur ions. Hydrogen molecules, H_2, may also play an important role here. It is difficult to estimate reliably the abundance of H_2 molecules in interstellar gas. The rates of the heating and cooling processes for H II regions are plotted in Fig. 6-5. The rates for cooling processes have been computed in

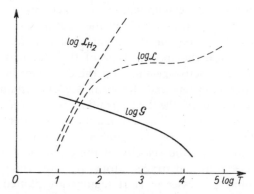

Figure 6-5. The curves of the heating and cooling rates, $\mathcal{G}$ and $\mathcal{L}$, in H I regions.

two versions: without the participation of H_2 molecules and on the assumption that H_2 molecules are ten times less numerous that hydrogen atoms. In both cases the curves intersect at a temperature of the order of several tens of degrees Kelvin.

When temperatures determined from measurements of spectral lines are compared with theoretical values calculated in the manner described above, they are found to agree for H II regions. In the case of H I regions, however, the observed temperatures are higher than the calculated values and amount to about 100°K. This indicates that the un-ionized hydrogen is heated by other factors than the radiation of stars. The collision of clouds and the interaction with cosmic radiation play a major role in heating these regions.

Section 63   Condensation of Interstellar Gas

As we know from the preceding Chapter, interstellar matter is the stuff out of which stars are made. Let us consider how initially scattered matter can concentrate into a condensation with a density many times the original value. The earliest stage in the evolution of a star is that of gravitational contraction. The star reduces its volume under its own gravitational forces. The low temperature and the attendant low pressures in the stellar interior are incapable of halting this process, until the nuclear reactions are ignited. However, will every gas condensation behave in this way? When a slight condensation is produced in air, as we know, propagation of a sound wave results. The gravitational forces with which gas molecules of small mass interact, are too small to be able to keep fast-moving gas molecules within the initial volume. The gravitational interactions become increasingly strong as we go over to larger and larger condensations. When the condensation formed exceeds a certain size

$$\lambda = \pi \sqrt{\frac{V_s^2}{\pi G \varrho}} \tag{6-19}$$

(where V_s is the speed of sound, and ϱ is the density of the medium), it will not disintegrate but will grow; it then enters the stage of self-gravitational contraction.

Let us evaluate the size of such a self-gravitational condensation which could be formed in interstellar matter. The mean density of interstellar gas is 1 atom/cm³. The velocity of sound is given by

$$V_s = \sqrt{\frac{\mathscr{R}T}{\mu}}, \tag{6-20}$$

where $\mathscr{R}$ is the gas constant in this formula. In H I regions V_s is about 1 km/sec and in H II regions is a dozen-odd km/sec. Taking a value of about 3 km/sec for the mean velocity of sound in the interstellar gas, we get $\lambda = 0.5$ kpc. The mass of such a condensation is

$$\mathfrak{M} \sim \lambda^3 \varrho \sim \frac{V_s^3}{G^{\frac{3}{2}} \varrho^{\frac{1}{2}}} \sim 10^{39} \text{ g} \sim 5 \times 10^5 \mathfrak{M}_\odot. \tag{6-21}$$

It is thus seen that the masses of self-gravitational condensations which could be formed directly out of interstellar matter are hundreds of thousands of times larger than stellar masses. Thus, the process of self-gravitational contraction of clouds of interstellar gas cannot directly lead to the formation of young stars. In order for self-gravitating condensations of solar mass to be formed in some medium, the density of that medium would have to be much greater than the mean density of the interstellar gas or else the temperature must be much lower. Therefore, a necessary condition for the formation of a star is that there occur processes leading to condensation of small interstellar clouds to a state from which self-gravitational contraction could proceed.

We do not know much about the mechanisms of such processes. Perhaps the initial condensation of matter is caused by a pressure difference which might be set up at the border between H I and H II regions building up about a hot star. When a bright star is born inside an un-ionized cloud (note that the formation time of massive type-*O* and type-*B* stars is shorter than the lifetime of the cloud), or if such a star happens by chance to pass through the cloud, it will begin to ionize the gas around it. The temperature of the gas being ionized increases about a hundredfold. The pressure of the gas will then rise about two-hundredfold (why?). A pressure jump appears at the boundary between the neutral ionized medium, and in consequence the ionized gas will begin to expand, pushing before it layers of neutral gas which are compressed more and more.

The rate at which such a shock wave propagates depends on the density of the medium. The fluctuations which occur in the density of the neutral gas may cause the condensed layer to break up into separate condensations surrounded by ionized gas. Figure 6-6 shows a schematic diagram of the

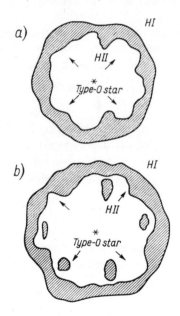

Figure 6-6. The formation of dense H I condensations (hatched areas) inside an expanding H II region.

development of an H II region around a hot star in a medium of non-uniform density: the moving ionization front refracts at places of increased density (Fig. 6-6a) and subsequently dense H I regions are surrounded by the ionized medium (Fig. 6-6b).

Under the high pressure of the ionized gas, such condensations fall inwards and perhaps the density inside them increases to such an extent that further contraction occurs under only their own gravitational forces.

Section 64   The Distribution and Motion of Interstellar Matter
in the Galaxy

With the development of radio engineering, it became possible for
astronomy to observe distant regions of our Galaxy and to investigate the
distribution of interstellar gas in it. Observations of the 21-cm line emitted
by neutral hydrogen has proved particularly fruitful. A catalogue of this
line measured in various directions in the Galaxy has been compiled on

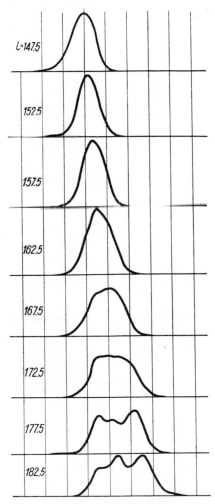

Figure 6-7. The profiles of the 21-cm line measured in the plane of the
Milky Way at intervals of 5° for galactic longitudes from 147°.5 to 182°.5
[On the basis of Muller and Westerhout, *Bull. Astron. Inst. Netherlands*
XIII, 151 (1957)].

the basis of these observations. Examples of the profiles of the 21-cm line measured in radiation arriving from several directions in the plane of the Galaxy are shown in Fig. 6-7.

We see that the profiles in Fig. 6-7 differ from each other in regard to both shape and number of peaks. The separation of peaks in one profile indicate that the radiation from this direction comes from several gaseous regions moving at different velocities with respect to the observer. By measuring the displacement of the peaks from the standard position of the 21-cm line, we can calculate the radial velocities of particular regions of gas from the Doppler effect. The method described in Sec. 57 can then be used to find the distribution of the rotational velocity of the Galaxy as

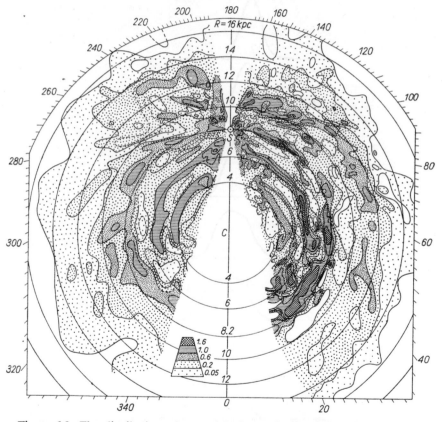

Figure 6-8. The distribution of neutral hydrogen in the Galaxy from observation in the 21-cm line, in atoms/cm³ (8.2 kpc has been taken as the distance from the Sun to the Galactic centre in constructing this diagram; a better value for this distance has now been determined to be about 10 kpc) [After Kerr, *MN RAS* **123**, 327 (1962)].

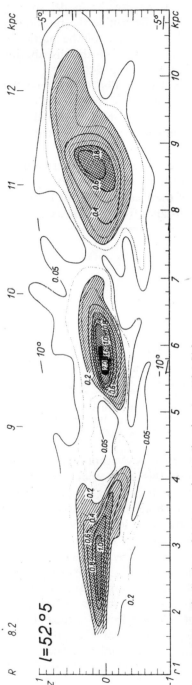

Figure 6-9. The distribution of hydrogen in the direction $l = 52°.5$ [After Muller and Westerhout, *Bull. Astron. Inst. Netherlands* **XIII**, 201 (1957)].

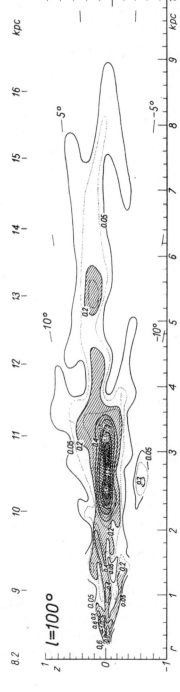

Figure 6-10. Distribution of hydrogen in the direction $l = 100°$ [After Muller and Westerhout, *Bull. Astron. Inst. Netherlands* **XIII**, 201 (1957)].

a function of the distance from the centre. If we use the model so constructed for the rotation of the Galaxy, we can determine the position of
gaseous regions which are responsible for the emission of the particular
peaks in the line profile. By such procedure we establish the distribution
of neutral hydrogen in the plane of the Milky Way (Fig. 6-8).

The spiral structure of the Galaxy is evident in Fig. 6-8. Interstellar
hydrogen concentrates in regions lying along spirals or circles girdling the
centre of the Galaxy. The spiral structure in the distribution of hydrogen
is also visible in Figs. 6-9 and 6-10 which present the density distribution
in planes perpendicular to the plane of the Galaxy.

From Figs. 6-8, 6-9, 6-10 we see that the mean density of the gas in the
spiral arms is 1 to 2 atoms/cm^3, whereas it decreases to 0.1 atom/cm^3 or
less between the spirals. The distribution of the mean density of hydrogen
is plotted in Fig. 6-11 as a function of the distance from the Galaxy centre.

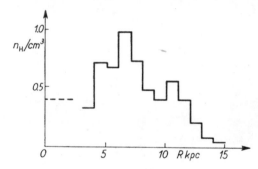

Figure 6-11. Distribution of the mean density of hydrogen as a function
of the distance to the centre of the Galaxy [After Muller and Westerhout, *Bull. Astron. Inst. Netherlands* **XIII**, 201 (1957)].

Almost the entire mass of the interstellar gas is concentrated in a thin
disk around the plane of the Galaxy. Does this mean that beyond this
layer there is no gas at all at considerable distances from the plane of the
Galaxy? Of course, this is not the case. Interstellar lines—above all of
calcium—have been detected in the spectra of stars observed at large
galactic latitudes. This indicates that interstellar gas, of much lower density,
also exists beyond the plane of the Milky Way. This gas, which forms the
galactic corona, is attracted by the matter in the galactic disk. It is thus
necessary to present a mechanism capable of maintaining the corona in
its present state. Two possibilities exist *a priori*: 1) the corona is in hydrostatic equilibrium, 2) strong turbulent motions exist in the corona. In the
first case, however, the gas temperature necessary for the pressure to
balance the attraction of the disk is very high (of the order of one million
Kelvin degrees). The second model seems more probable. According to

it, the corona would be sustained by strong turbulent motions of gas and clouds ejected from the disk at high velocities. A major role could be played by the pressure of turbulent magnetic fields acting strongly on the sparse coronal medium.

Section 65   Instellar Polarization of Stellar Light and the Magnetic
             Field in the Galaxy

Interesting information about the interstellar medium is provided by observations of the polarization of stellar light. Figures 6-12 and 6-13 show the results of measurements of polarization of light from stars observed in directions perpendicular (Fig. 6-12) and parallel (Fig. 6-13) to a spiral arm of the Galaxy.

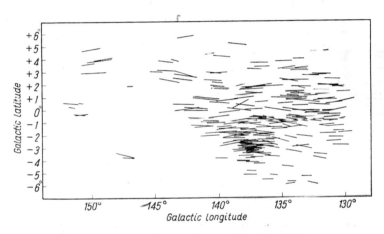

Figure 6-12. The polarization of the light from stars observed perpendicular to the spiral arm (the length of the segments indicated in the drawing is proportional to the degree of polarization; their direction coincides with that of the maximum vibrations of the electric vector) [After Hiltner, *Astrophys. Journ. Suppl. Ser.* **II**, 389 (1956)].

As we look at Fig. 6-12, we are struck by the fact that the light from almost all stars is polarized in one direction, approximately parallel to the plane of the Galaxy. This indicates that the polarization must take place in the interstellar medium since we cannot indicate any agent which could cause stars remote from each other to radiate light polarized in the same plane.* The existence of a correlation between the polarization and interstellar reddening also points to the interstellar origin of the polarization.

---

* This does not, of course, mean that in this way we completely exclude the possibility of the stars themselves emitting polarized light; on the contrary, stars which send out polarized radiation do indeed exist.

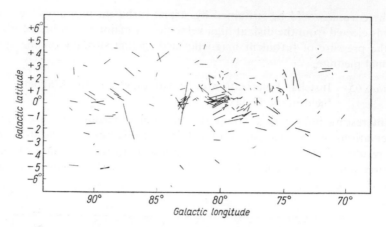

Figure 6-13. The polarization of the light from stars observed parallel to the spiral arm [After Hiltner, *Astrophys. Journ. Suppl. Ser.* **II**, 389 (1956)].

The directions of polarization are distributed chaotically in Fig. 6-13 as we look along the spiral arm of the Galaxy. Comparison of Figs. 6-12 and 6-13 indicates that the influence of the agent causing polarization is different when we look in different directions. It will be our task to find such an agent which could provide an explanation for the phenomenon.

The observed polarization of light in the interstellar medium could be due only to scattering from nonspherical grains of dust. If the dust grains in interstellar space were oriented so as to line up with their long or short axis parallel to some preferred direction, we might expect natural (unpolarized) light to be polarized when passing through that medium. This would be due to the fact that scattering from dust grains would attenuate the vibrations of the electric vector component parallel to the long axes of the grains more than the component parallel to the short axes of the grains. Upon passing through the medium, the components of the electric vector vibrations would not be equal to each other; the light would be partially polarized parallel to the direction of the short axes of the grains. The fact that they have a particular orientation does not mean the grains of dust are not moving, especially rotating about an axis passing through their centre. However, in the event of rotational motion of the grains, their axes of rotation should display a tendency towards ordering.

Since radiation travelling in the plane of the Galaxy perpendicular to a spiral arm is polarized in a direction parallel to the Galaxy plane (Fig. 6-12), the short axes of the dust grains should be parallel to that plane. Light from stars observed as we look along a spiral arm (Fig. 6-13) are only slightly polarized and the directions of polarization are distributed chaotically. This indicates that the projections of the long axes of the dust grains are distributed at random in a plane perpendicular to the arm. Since the short axes of the dust grains lie in directions in the plane of the Galaxy, and the projections of the long axes are scattered at random in the plane perpendicular to the spiral arm, the short axes of the dust grains must tend to line up along the spiral arm.

As a result of collisions with atoms in the medium and with each other, the dust grains will be set into rotation and at the same time their ordering will be destroyed; thus, if the ordering is to be preserved, some agent must be continually causing the dust grains to align themselves with their short axes parallel to the direction of the spiral arm. The rotating dust grain will tend to rotate about its shortest axis (the axis of largest moment of inertia). Thus, the agent responsible for the ordering of the dust grains is one capable of lining up the rotation axes of the grains parallel to the spiral arm.

A magnetic field parallel to the spiral arm could be such an agent. If we assume that some admixtures (of the order of 10%) of metal are constituents of the dust, the grain will be capable of magnetization by an external magnetic field. The magnetization of the grain will result in a magnetic moment which causes the rotation axis of the grain to precess. Owing to the rotation, the grain of dust continually changes its position with respect to the external magnetic field, and this necessitates remagnetization of the grain. The energy used up in remagnetizing the grain comes from the kinetic energy of the rotating grain itself. As a result of the loss of kinetic energy, the axis of rotation of the grain describes about the direction of the magnetic field a cone of precession with an ever decreasing angular opening (just as the axis of a spinning top, which loses energy through friction against the base, describes about the vertical a cone of precession with a decreasing apex angle). This process will lead to the grains lining up with their small axes (axes of rotation) in the direction of the magnetic field.

This mechanism of orientation of the dust grains provides a good explanation for the observations of polarization described at the beginning of this section. According to this mechanism, the magnetic field is directed along the spiral arms of the Galaxy. The strength of the magnetic field in the Galaxy in the neighbourhood of the Sun, evaluated on the basis of other considerations as well, is of the order of $10^{-5}-10^{-6}$ Oe.

The interaction of the magnetic field with interstellar matter no doubt plays an important role in many phenomena occurring in the Galaxy and may perhaps even exert a vital influence on the distribution of this matter in the plane of the Galaxy.

Chapter 7 Extra-galactic Astronomy

GALAXIES

The preceding two chapters were devoted to a discussion of the structure of our Galaxy. The Galaxy is representative of a numerous group of astronomical objects—galaxies, each of which is made up of thousands of millions of stars linked together by their mutual gravitational interaction. Studies of galaxies, tracking of the motions of stars and interstellar matter inside them, and observations of phenomena occurring in them make for a better understanding of the structure of our Galaxy and discovery of typical processes which are decisive in regard to the evolution of our Galaxy. At the same time, observations of galaxies provide a starting point for conclusions about the structure of the Universe as a whole.

Section 66   Types, Masses, Sizes, and Distances of Galaxies

The two nearest galaxies, called the Large and Small Magellanic Clouds (Cf. Plates 27 and 28), which are visible to the unaided eye from the southern hemisphere, are at a distance of about 50–60 kpc from us. These are objects with masses much smaller (by a factor of several tens) than our Galaxy and their diameters are about 25 and 10 pc, respectively. The Magellanic Clouds have been observed to contain a large number of star clusters, individual stars of various types, as well as interstellar matter, in the form of both luminous clouds of ionized hydrogen and neutral hydrogen detected by radio observations. Measurements of the radial velocities of objects belonging to the Magellanic Clouds indicate the clouds are rotating. In view of the short distance from the Galaxy and the low radial velocity (about 40 km/sec for the Large Cloud and 15 km/sec for the Small Cloud) with respect to the Galactic centre, it would seem that the Magellanic Clouds are satellites of our Galaxy, permanently bound to it by gravitational interactions.

Our Galaxy and the Magellanic Clouds comprise part of the Local Group. This is a group of about twenty galaxies contained in a region about 500 kpc in size. A possible physical connection between the galaxies in the Local Group might be indicated by the fact that the nearest galaxy external to this Group lies at a distance of about 1.5 Mpc.

A galaxy in Andromeda, which is the brightest galaxy in the northern skies, also belongs to the Local Group. It is probably similar to our Galaxy in structure. It also has distinct spiral arms, with a high content of gas and dust, in which we observe a considerable number of bright stars of the early spectral types (Cf. Plate 29). It has a diameter of about 30–40 kpc. Near the Andromeda Galaxy, called the Great Nebula of Andromeda, we can see two galaxies (elliptical-shaped in photographs) which no doubt form a triple system with it.

The visible shape of galaxies constitutes a basis for their classification into types. The following basic types of galaxies are distinguished: elliptical galaxies E (Plate 30), lens-shaped type SO (Plate 31), spiral S (Plate 32), and irregular I (Plate 33).

When giving the type of an elliptical galaxy, we usually specify the degree of its flattening (ellipticity) on a scale from 0 to 7; the number specifying the flattening is

$$ n = 10 \left(1 - \frac{b}{a} \right), \qquad (7\text{-}1) $$

where a and b denote the observed angular dimensions of the major and minor axes, respectively, of the galaxy. Thus, an elliptical galaxy of axis ratio $b/a = 0.4$ is designated as an E 6 galaxy. Galaxies with an ellipticity of more than $\frac{a-b}{a} = 0.7$ have not been observed.

Type $S0$ and S galaxies are divided into two groups, according to the classification introduced by Hubble. One of them comprises galaxies in which a distinct concentration of stars is observed about a straight line which lies in the plane of the galaxy and passes through the centre of that galaxy; we call these barred spirals and denote them by symbols $SB0$ and SB, respectively. Spiral galaxies are further differentiated according to the size and regularity of the structure of their spiral arms; this is done by adding a lower case letter to the type symbol of the galaxy: a (for galaxies with the least distinct structure of spirals), b, c, or d (for galaxies in which the spiral arms are very distinct). Plate 34 shows $S0$ and S galaxies. Frequently when referring to some group of galaxies, we give only those symbols which describe the given group. For instance, in writing S we have in mind all spiral galaxies, regardless of whether they are barred spirals or not.

It is extremely difficult to determine galaxian* distances. This is so first and foremost because in many galaxies we cannot distinguish individual stars which could serve as a basis for estimating galaxian distances. But even in cases when we can do this, the stars are in general very faint and this in turn affects the accuracy of the results. If we can detect cepheids

---

* Galaxian refers to extra-galactic systems in contrast to galactic which refers to our Galaxy, the Milky Way.

in the given galaxy, we determine their absolute magnitude (Cf. Sec. 43) from measurements of the period of variations in their luminosity. We then calculate the distance to the given galaxy by using the formula

$$M-m = -5\log r+5-A, \tag{7-2}$$

where A is the interstellar extinction in the Galaxy (estimated e.g. from observations of stars in our Galaxy which lie far from its plane, beyond the layer of interstellar matter, in the direction of the galaxy under observation). Formula (7-2) can be used whenever we can evaluate the absolute magnitude of at least one star within the given galaxy, Above all, bright stars of types O and B (apart from cepheids) are such stars. The situation is advantageous when a nova is observed within the given galaxy and variations in its luminosity can be followed. As we know from Sec. 43, the absolute magnitude of a nova at maximum luminosity is related to the rate at which is brightness decreases after the explosion. Thus, observations of the brightness of a nova at the time of its explosion and for some time after provide information about the absolute magnitude of the nova. Finally, observations of supernovae may serve to evaluate galaxian distances, especially in relation to galaxies which are so remote that fainter stars cannot be distinguished within them. However, this method of determining the distances to galaxies on the basis of observations of member stars can be applied only to the nearest galaxies.

In the case of galaxies in which individual stars are not distinguishable, distances may be gauged by measurements of the total luminosity of galaxies. As in the case of stars, we can define (Cf. Sec. 45) the absolute and apparent magnitudes of galaxies as measures, respectively, of the amount of energy emitted by the entire galaxy in a unit time and of the illumination from that galaxy. It turns out that the absolute luminosities of galaxies are associated with their types. The absolute luminosities of galaxies can be calculated by Eq. (7-2) on the basis of observations of near galaxies, whose distances may be determined by the methods described above (e.g. by observation of cepheids). For this purpose, of course, the apparent magnitudes of the galaxies must replace m in Eq. (7-2). Comparison of the calculated absolute luminosities with the types of the galaxies serves to determine the correlation between these quantities. Assuming further that this same relation between type and magnitude holds for remote galaxies, we can estimate the magnitudes of galaxies on the basis of types.

The relation between absolute luminosity and galaxy type is tested additionally on more distant objects which we are justified in assuming to be all at the same distance. This condition is satisfied by galaxies belonging to clusters. A more precise examination leads us to the conclusion that the distribution of galaxies on the celestial sphere is not exactly uniform; the density of galaxies is observed to be higher in some places than in others. An explanation for this effect may be that in the given direction at some distance from the observer there is a cluster of galaxies which, being projected upon the celestial sphere, is detected as a local increase in the number of galaxies per unit surface area. The limits and sizes of clusters of galaxies are not so sharply defined as those of star clusters, but an unquestionable concentration of galaxies in some areas may be detected by statistical analysis of galaxy counts. Thus, even if we do not know the distance to a cluster accurately, but merely know that this distance is much larger than the size of the cluster, we may then assume that all of its member galaxies are at approximately the same distance from us. The right-hand side of Eq. (7-2) will then be the same for all of these galaxies and, hence, the absolute magnitudes of the galaxies in the cluster can be obtained by adding a constant (the same for all members of the cluster) to the apparent magnitudes. For this reason, in the case of the members of the cluster, the correlation between the absolute magnitude and type of a galaxy should be transformed into an apparent magnitude-galaxy type relation which can be checked directly by observation.

After this analysis it turns out (Cf. Table 7-1) that Sb galaxies are among the brightest while elliptical galaxies, and above all irregular galaxies, are less bright than the spiral types and that the absolute magnitudes of galaxies differ considerably (by more than 1^m) within one and the same type.

TABLE 7-1

Relation Between Galaxy Type and Mean Absolute Magnitude

Type	E	S0	Sa	Sb	Sc	Sd	I
M	$-18^m.6$	$-18^m.7$	$-18^m.9$	$-19^m.0$	$-18^m.9$	$-18^m.5$	$-16^m.5$

Thus, if we know the type of a galaxy, we can evaluate its absolute magnitude and then, after measuring its apparent magnitude, go on to use Eq. (7-2) to determine its distance. This method may, however, lead to a considerable error in the evaluation of distances in cases when the magnitude of the given galaxy differs from the mean value for the given type. A very rough estimate of the distance can also be made for very remote clusters in which it would be extremely difficult to determine the types of galaxies observed. In this case, the assumption is made that, say, the fifth brightest galaxy in the cluster has the same absolute magnitude in all clusters. This method, however, is of low accuracy and is used when all other methods fail.

A method employed very frequently to determine galaxian distances is one based on Hubble's law which will be discussed in the next section.

The masses of galaxies are in general found by dynamic methods. One of them consists in measuring the radial velocities of the members of a binary galactic system. This method utilizes Kepler's third law. In order to apply it, we must know the semimajor axis of the relative orbit of the galaxies in the system, that is, we must previously find the distance of the system and the angular distance of the members of the system. Moreover, we must make an additional assumption concerning the inclination of the orbit to the line-of-sight and concerning the current position of the bodies in the orbit. Another, more accurate method (which may also be used for single galaxies) is to measure the velocities of stars (or the interstellar matter) within the galaxy under study. These velocities and their distribution along the radius of the galaxy depend on the distribution of mass within the galaxy. This method may be used successfully for galaxies of known distances and angular dimensions large enough for the velocities of stars in particular parts of the galaxy to be measurable.

The mass-luminosity relation of a galaxy is also frequently used to evaluate the mass. It turns out that the $\mathfrak{M}/L$ ratio depends on the type of galaxy and is highest for elliptical galaxies, decreasing as we proceed from spirals to irregulars. Thus, the mass of a galaxy may be found from its type and luminosity. Galaxian masses, evaluated by the methods mentioned above, are contained within the interval 10^8 to 10^{13} solar masses, the elliptical galaxies being the most massive and densest and the irregulars the least massive.

The dependence of the mass-luminosity ratio on the type of galaxy indicates that the relative abundance of stars of various types is not the same in all galaxies; namely, spiral galaxies contain many population-I stars whereas population II predominates in ellipticals. Galaxies also vary in regard to the content of interstellar matter. The strength of interstellar lines in galactic spectra increases as we go through the consecutive types of spiral galaxies towards the irregulars. The same is true of radio observations of un-ionized hydrogen.

We have thus far been discussing the types of so-called normal galaxies. However, there are a number of galaxies which differ considerably in structure from these normal galaxies. Galaxy M 82 (Cf. Plate 35), whose structure testifies to a recent explosion, is a representative example. Photographs of M 82 show massive jets of gas expelled along the shorter axis of the galaxy in both directions away from the galactic plane. Spectroscopic measurements of these jets indicate that they possess a velocity of the order of 1000 km/sec directed away from the centre of the galaxy, and the densities of the jets are of the order of 10 protons/cm^3. Hence, the mass determined for the jets amounts to 6×10^6 solar masses. The complicated structure of the jets suggests the existence of a relatively strong magnetic field in them. The emission of polarized radiation in a continuous spectrum by the jets could also indicate the presence of a magnetic field. This radiation, called synchrotron radiation, is produced because free electrons are subjected to accelerations due the to magnetic field. The fact that such relatively large masses in M 82 have such high velocities undoubtedly testifies to an explosion in the galactic nucleus. It is difficult at this time to give the reason for such an explosion or to state whether it is one of the evolutionary stages in the life of every galaxy.

Seyfert and N-type galaxies also belong to the category of peculiar galaxies. Seyfert galaxies have characteristic small (apparently points, star-like) but very bright nuclei. The outer parts of these galaxies, on the other hand, do not differ from normal $S0$-Sc types. The spectrum of light from the nuclei of Seyfert galaxies contains very strong emission lines of considerable width, which indicate that within these galaxies gases move chaotically at speeds of up to several thousand km/sec. In general, these galaxies are more powerful sources of radio emission than are normal spiral galaxies of comparable visual magnitudes. Seyfert galaxies have been observed to vary in all intervals of the spectrum, but there is no distinct coincidence in the variations of brightness at various wavelengths. Similar features are found in the radiation from N-type galaxies which are also characterized by small, bright nuclei but with no outer parts of these galaxies visible. Type-N galaxies are more distant than the Seyfert type but they may perhaps be objects of the same kind, only absolutely brighter (we see them at greater distances), whose outer parts (of lower surface luminosity) are not visible at such great distances. N-type galaxies are in general much brighter than normal types.

The dimensions of the luminous parts (nuclei) of Seyfert and N-type galaxies can be evaluated from a knowledge of the rate at which their luminosities vary. A major change in the luminosity (say by a factor of two) of any source of radiation cannot occur in less time than light requires to traverse the diameter of the source, since no factor causing a change in the brightness of the particular parts of the luminous region can travel faster than the speed of light; moreover, radiation received by an observer at a given instant was emitted by different parts of the source at various instants, depending on the distance of those parts from the observer. Thus, by observing the rate at which the luminosity of a source varies, we can give the upper limit of the allowable values of its diameter. Considerable variations of luminosity occurring within a week have been observed in the case of several N-type galaxies. The conclusion may therefore be that the nuclei of these objects must have a diameter of less (perhaps considerably less) than 0.06 pc. Thus, in comparison to galaxies these are extremely small objects, of dimensions rather close to that of the solar system (many periodic comets of the solar system move away from the Sun to distances of greater than 0.06 pc), emitting an energy higher than that released in thermonuclear processes in the interiors of all the stars of an average galaxy.

Section 67   Hubble's Law

A characteristic feature of the spectra of extragalactic objects is that all the spectral lines and bands are shifted towards the red. This effect is observed in all galaxies beyond the Local Group. The extent to which the spectral lines are displaced depends on the wavelength; for all lines in the spectrum of a given galaxy, the value of the ratio z, called the red shift, is constant (does not depend on λ),

$$z = \Delta\lambda/\lambda = \text{const}, \tag{7-3}$$

where $\Delta\lambda$ is the magnitude of the displacement of the line which normally corresponds to the wavelength λ. The constancy of this ratio, originally detected only in the visible region, was also confirmed for radio emission in the Fifties and it turned out that the values of this ratio are identical for radiation in the visible and radio regions.

Another observational fact is that a correlation exists between the red shift and the distances of galaxies studied (Cf. Plate 36). In 1929 Hubble demonstrated the relation

$$z = \frac{H}{c} r, \tag{7-4}$$

where r is the distance to the galaxy, c is the velocity of light, and H is a proportionality factor, called the Hubble constant. Equation (7-4) is satisfied statistically by all galaxies, but this does not mean that there are no random peculiar velocities of galaxies which also cause a displacement of spectral lines, hence somewhat altering the observed values of z, and are responsible for some deviations from Eq. (7-4) for individual objects. These deviations may completely conceal the Hubble effect in those cases when the values of z yielded by Eq. (7-4) are small, which is the case for near galaxies. This is why Hubble's law (law of the red shift) is not satisfied by the galaxies of the Local Group.

The only reason known at present for a spectral line displacement proportional to the wavelength is that the source of light is moving relative to the observer. Then, as follows from Doppler's law, (relativistic form)

$$z = \frac{\Delta\lambda}{\lambda} = \frac{1 + \dfrac{v}{c}}{\sqrt{1 - \dfrac{v^2}{c^2}}} - 1, \tag{7-5}$$

where v is the velocity of the source of light with respect to the observer.

Since $v \ll c$ for objects which are not very distant (and that is the type Hubble observed), we can use the formula in the simplified form

$$z = \frac{\Delta\lambda}{\lambda} \approx \frac{v}{c}. \tag{7-6}$$

Equations (7-4) and (7-6) yield

$$v = Hr, \tag{7-7}$$

which means that the velocities with which galaxies are moving away from us (velocities of recession) are proportional to the distances. Determinations of Hubble's constant give a value of $H \approx 100$ km/sec $\cdot$ Mpc. This means that a galaxy, say 10 Mpc from us, is moving away with a velocity of 1000 km/sec.

The recession of galaxies away from us according to the law given by Eq. (7-7) does not signify that our Galaxy is in any privileged position in the Universe since the same effect of galaxies moving away with velocities proportional to the distances would also be observed if the observer were placed in any arbitrary galaxy. Indeed, let us denote any two arbitrary galaxies by G_1 and G_2 (Cf. Fig. 7-1). Let r_1 and r_2 denote the vectors drawn from our Galaxy to galaxies G_1 and G_2, respectively. Thus, by Hubble's law the velocities v_1 and v_2 are given by

$$\mathbf{v}_1 = H\mathbf{r}_1 \quad \text{and} \quad \mathbf{v}_2 = H\mathbf{r}_2 \tag{7-8}$$

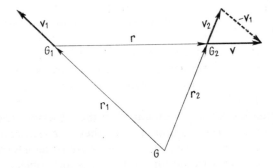

Figure 7-1. Hubble's Law and the position of the observer.

and, hence, the velocity $\mathbf{v}$ of galaxy G_2 relative to galaxy G_1 is proportional to the distance $\mathbf{r}$ between them

$$\mathbf{v} = \mathbf{v}_2 - \mathbf{v}_1 = H\mathbf{r}_2 - H\mathbf{r}_1 = H(\mathbf{r}_2 - \mathbf{r}_1) = H\mathbf{r}. \tag{7-9}$$

The fact that the red shift is proportional to the distances of the galaxies is exploited to evaluate the distances to those objects. Indeed, the value of z is frequently given instead of the distance for remote galaxies.

Section 68   Quasars

One of the greatest astronomical discoveries of the past decade has been the detection of quasars (quasi-stellar radio sources). This happened in the course of identifying radio sources with objects observed in the visual region. It turns out that some radio sources can be identified with objects whose optical images, just as those of stars, are point images. It seemed that here we had a new type of object—stars radiating very powerful radio emission, much more intense than the radiation of normal stars. More accurate information about the nature of these objects could be provided by spectroscopic study of their spectra. But here very serious difficulties were encountered. The spectra obtained were not similar to those of any known star. It was not until 1963 that four strong emission lines in the spectrum of an object designated by the symbol 3C273 were identified as the Balmer series hydrogen lines $H_\beta - H_\varepsilon$ with a red shift of $z = 0.158$. (The symbol 3C273 consists of the abbreviation of the catalogue name—third Cambridge catalogue of radio sources and of the number of the source in that catalogue—273).

Such a large red shift for a stellar-like object has very far-reaching consequences. If we had continued to treat quasars as radio stars occurring in our Galaxy, the only explanation for such a large red shift would be to assume that quasars had extremely large masses and very high densities. As emerges from the theory of relativity, the spectrum of radiation emitted in a strong gravitational field experiences a red shift. In order to explain such large observed values of z we would have to assume, for instance, that quasars of a mass comparable to that of the Sun have a radius of the order of 10 km. This is contradicted, however, by some observational results. A number of so-called forbidden lines, i.e. lines which can occur only in gases of low densities, have been identified in the spectra of quasars. These facts induce us to reject the hypothesis that quasars are radio stars belonging to our Galaxy.

Thus, another explanation remains for the observed red shift in the spectra of quasars: the assumption that they are extragalactic objects. If the large values of z observed for quasars were to be interpreted according to Hubble's law, they would turn out to be distant objects. For instance, the distance calculated from Eq. (7-4) for 3C273 is about 500 Mpc. At present we know some 200 objects of this type, and the largest observed value of z is about 2.9, which would correspond to recession at 0.88 of the speed of light. These would thus be the most distant objects we observe. This would necessitate the assumption that these objects are extremely bright. Indeed, quasars would be the brightest objects observed in the Universe. Thus, the absolute magnitude calculated from Eq. (7-2) for 3C273 ($m = 13^m$) is -25^m, which means an emission of energy at a rate of the order of 10^{45} ergs per second. On the basis of present data we cannot determine what processes could be responsible for such abundant production of energy in quasars nor can we say what factors could have led to the formation of these objects.

The energy distribution in the spectra of quasars is different from that in the spectra of normal galaxies. In comparison to normal galaxies, they display an excess of radiation in the ultraviolet (this property enables quasars to be detected and distinguished from galaxies by photometric examination), and 3C273 has been identified as a source of X-rays. The intensity of radiation in the ultraviolet part of the spectrum decreases in inverse proportion to the frequency and is polarized to the extent of several per cent, which can be explained on the basis of the theory of synchrotron radiation. This means that what we have here is the glowing of fast-moving electrons in a strong magnetic field. The bulk of the energy is in general emitted in the infrared part of the spectrum. Spectral lines are observed, both emission lines produced by hot gaseous regions and absorption lines. In a number of cases, it has been found that there are several arrays of lines which display different red shifts. This may be due to absorption of radiation by clouds of interstellar gas *en route* between the quasar and the observer or else by clouds ejected at high speed by the quasar itself.

The intensity of quasar radiation, in both the optical and the radio regions, undergoes fluctuation. In some cases major changes of luminosity are relatively rapid since they take place within a period of a few weeks. This is undoubtedly an argument in favour of the view that these objects (or at least their luminous parts) are very small. This fact was indicated by the very first optical observations inasmuch as images of quasars appeared as stellar images in photographs. The use of radio interferometers with a base length of the order of thousands of kilometres (hence, with suitably high resolving power) made it possible to determine that the angular diameters of quasars do not exceed 0.001 second of arc.

The search for quasars by photometric methods utilizing their great brightness in the ultraviolet led to the discovery of a number of objects similar to quasars except for emitting radio-frequency radiation. Since these objects, just as quasars and stars, are imaged as points, they were named quasi-stellar objects, QSO for short. Just as quasars, they exhibit a large red shift, an excess of ultraviolet radiation, a continuous spectrum with an appearance characteristic of synchrotron radiation, and a high power of radiation—of the order of 10^{45} ergs/sec. Thus, we have every reason to believe that these objects are of the same type as quasars, or, in other words, that quasars are radio-emitting QSO's.

The number of radio-quiet QSO's observed is less than the number of quasars discovered. Undoubtedly what is involved here is an observational selection effect in that many quasars are powerful radio sources and, therefore, can be detected with relative ease in the radio-frequency region, whereas radio-quiet QSO's are relatively faint objects in the sky in the visible region. Some information about the true ratio of the number of quasars to all QSO's may be provided by a more accurate count of these objects in small areas of the sky, small enough so that it is possible to study all objects up to a particular observed magnitude. Counts of this kind lead us to the conclusion that perhaps quasars constitute less than 1% of the total number of QSO's.

The similarity of the nuclei of Seyfert galaxies, N-type galaxies, and QSO's, namely the unusually small size, the excess of ultraviolet radiation as compared to normal galaxies, fluctuations in luminosity and high power of radiation (although different for the various types of these objects— least for Seyfert galaxies, most for QSO's) allows us to make the supposition that (without going into the nature of these processes) all of these objects have a common mechanism of energy production. However, the efficiency of this mechanism differs for these objects and, consequently, Seyfert galaxies are observable only when relatively close to the observer, whereas QSO's are observed even when very distant (hence, the great values of z measured for many of these objects).

COSMOLOGY

As science and technology develop, the region accessible to astronomical instruments is extended, astronomical observations reach out towards increasingly distant objects, and we come to know more and more of the Universe. At the same time, there remains the question: what is the nature of the Universe as a whole? What is its evolution—past and future? The answer to these questions requires a generalization of the results obtained by observation, first and foremost in the realm of extragalactic astronomy, as well as extrapolation to the entire Universe of the laws of physics confirmed experimentally or observationally for phenomena which are of finite duration and occur in a bounded region. This extrapolation provides opportunities for constructing various theoretical models of the Universe, which would be acceptable from the point of view of the present state of the art in physics and could subsequently be compared with observations. Only observational confirmation of one of the theoretical models of the Universe, coupled with simultaneous demonstration that all the others are incompatible with the results of observations, could completely resolve the fundamental problem of cosmology: the problem of the structure of the Universe.

Section 69 The Cosmological Principle

Generalization of the results of extragalactic astronomy obtained by observation requires assumptions as to the possibility of treating the known part of the Universe as representative of the entire Universe. In other words, the starting point for conclusions about the structure of the Universe is the assumption that the part we know does not differ in regard to its cardinal features from the other parts which are inaccessible to our observations. This assumption, known as the cosmological principle, may be formulated as follows: knowledge of the Universe does not depend on the position of the observer, i.e. regardless of the position of the observer, the image of the Universe surrounding him is the same.

A consequence of the cosmological principle is the assumption that matter in the Universe is distributed in a uniform manner. Of course, the question may arise as to what should uniformity of distribution of matter mean. This concept can certainly not be used in reference to the distribution of stars; stars are grouped in galaxies. Similarly, we cannot speak of uniform distribution of galaxies; these (at least, some of them) are concentrated in clusters of galaxies. Consequently, the concept of uniformity should be applied to the distribution of clusters of galaxies providing, of course, that it does not turn out in the future that they tend to associate in clusters of a higher order.

Note that the effect of galaxies receding with velocities proportional to the distance, as described by Hubble's law, is in accordance with the essence of the cosmological principle.

The cosmological principle will not be fully verifiable by observation as long as we are unable to observe the entire Universe (if this will ever be possible). We can nevertheless treat it as the simplest working assumption, necessary in order to construct cosmological models.

A natural extension of the above weak cosmological principle is the so-called perfect cosmological principle, employed by some astronomers, which can be formulated as follows: regardless of the position of the observer and the instant at which he makes the observation, the image of the Universe around him is the same. Thus, according to the perfect cosmological principle, the image of the Universe does not depend on time; in particular, the density of matter in the Universe does not vary. This can be made to agree with the observed general recession of the galaxies (causing the mean density to decrease) only if new matter is assumed to be created continuously. The perfect cosmological principle does not, however, contradict the principle of conservation of mass (or mass and energy) since the creation of new matter postulated by the perfect cosmological principle is very slow (about 2 atoms of hydrogen per km^3 in a year) and, hence, is completely undetectable in the laboratory by present-day experimental techniques.

Section 70   Cosmological Models

The objective of cosmological models is to give the relations between the functions which characterize the Universe as a whole and to present the time-dependence of these functions. Some of these functions are: the mean density $\varrho(t)$ of matter and the scale factor $R(t)$ given by the formula

$$\mathbf{r} = R(t)\mathbf{r}_0, \tag{7-10}$$

where $\mathbf{r}$ and $\mathbf{r}_0$, respectively, denote the present and initial position (at some instant t_0) of any arbitrary galaxy (neglecting its peculiar motion with respect to its neighbours) in a reference frame fixed at some arbitrary point (e.g. our Galaxy).

Of course, by the cosmological principle $R(t)$ is the same for all galaxies and does not depend on the reference frame. Moreover,

$$R(t_0) = 1. \tag{7-11}$$

The function $R(t)$ describes the expansion or contraction of the Universe. It is related to Hubble's constant, since

$$\mathbf{v} = \frac{d\mathbf{r}}{dt} = \frac{dR}{dt}\,\mathbf{r}_0 = R^{-1}\frac{dR}{dt}\,(R\mathbf{r}_0) = R^{-1}\frac{dR}{dt}\,\mathbf{r}. \tag{7-12}$$

Thus, if we confine ourselves to near objects, we have the relation

$$\frac{1}{R(t_1)}\frac{dR(t_1)}{dt} = H, \tag{7-13}$$

where t_1 denotes the present instant of time.

The dependence of the function R on the time t is determined by differential equations describing the motion of the system under the influence of the interactions occurring within it. The strongest of all interactions governing large-scale motions in the Universe are the gravitational interactions. Thus, the problem of the structure of the Universe is bound up with the problem of the theory of the gravitational field, and constructing a cosmological model consists in solving the differential equations of the gravitational field with appropriate initial conditions and values of the parameters appearing in these equations.

To consider the various cosmological models would be beyond the scope of this book. We shall merely mention one class of cosmological models, the so-called relativistic models of the Universe. They constitute an interesting group because they relate the density $\varrho(t)$ of matter and the scale factor $R(t)$ to the geometry of space. Namely, according to the theory of relativity the paths of light quanta (particles endowed with energy and, hence, mass) are curved in the presence of a gravitational field. This effect has been confirmed by observations during total eclipses of the Sun when it was found that the position of stars near the solar limb are somewhat displaced from the Sun with respect to their normal position in the celestial sphere. The curvature of the paths traversed by light can be treated as the existence of curvature of space itself in which radiation propagates along the shortest lines between the source of light and the observer. In this sense, space in which light travels in straight lines, is space of zero curvature or Euclidean space. The theory of relativity, therefore, allows the existence of models of the Universe with nonvanishing curvature, positive or negative.

In models of the Universe constructed only on the basis of the weak cosmological principle and the principle of conservation of mass, the function $R(t)$ is related to the density of matter. In these models, the general expansion of the galaxies is accompanied by a decrease in the mean density of matter at every point in the Universe. Conversely, in models utilizing the perfect cosmological principle, the density remains unchanged, despite the existing expansion of the Universe.

Individual cosmological models envisage other relations between quantities which are directly observable. Comparison of these relations with observations may provide a basis for choosing a model which corresponds to reality.

Section 71   Observational Tests

The principal factor permitting a choice of cosmological model is that the evolution of the Universe proceeds in a different way in each model. Use is made here of the fact that the electromagnetic radiation reaching us at present was emitted by the source at some time in the past. For this reason, regions of the Universe which are at various distances from us are seen at different stages of evolution. However, in order to be able to resolve the question of the evolution of the Universe by observational means, and hence to choose an appropriate model, we must reach out to very distant objects, so distant in fact that the light from them travels for a time over which major evolutionary changes may take place. This compels us to study very faint objects and this in turn entails formidable observational difficulties.

One of the relations employed to test cosmological models is the red shift-magnitude relation. Hubble's law states that for not very distant objects, (those for which we could measure the red shift and distance independently), the red shift and distance are proportional to each other. If we were to observe very distant objects, however, we could expect deviations from proportionality. These deviations would be the result of a different rate of expansion of the Universe in the past. For this reason, study of the red shift-distance relation could serve for choosing an appropriate cosmological model. However, difficulties are encountered here in measuring the distances of very distant objects (Cf. Sec. 66). The apparent magnitude of galaxies is a directly measured quantity which subsequently serves to evaluate the distance. Hence, in testing cosmological models, use is frequently made of the red shift-apparent magnitude relation instead of the theoretical distance-red shift relation obtained directly from cosmological models. The transition from the first of these relations to the second, however, requires several assumptions and is hindered by a number of additional effects. Namely, the measurement of the distance to very remote objects is based in the many cases on the adoption of some absolute magnitude for one of the brightest galaxies in the cluster. We may, however, encounter a selection effect whereby we observe only galaxy-abundant clusters. Distant ones, with few stars, may escape detection when we observe the faintest galaxies perceivable. But the absolute magnitudes of the brightest galaxies in large clusters may be smaller (in magnitudes, which corresponds to brighter galaxies) than in smaller clusters. For this reason the distances to remote clusters might be systematically over-estimated. Moreover, any extinction in the intergalaxian matter would undermine the assumed relation between the absolute and apparent magnitude and the distance to the galaxies. Another effect is that of the red shift of the galactic spectra which causes the luminosity of distant galaxies to be measured in a different part of the spectrum than the luminosity of near galaxies. Finally, various cosmological models postulate that the evolution of galaxies has a different influence on their mean brightness in some region. For instance, in models of the Universe which assume the principle of conservation of mass, the average age of the observed galaxies may increase with time. Because of evolutionary changes of the galaxies themselves, the more distant seem to be younger than the nearer ones, and the absolute magnitude of galaxies may depend on their age. It is a different matter in the case of models assuming the perfect cosmological principle. In this case, we have young galaxies being formed continuously out of new matter that is created continuously. Thus, the distribution of galaxies according to their age does not vary in each region of the Universe. By virtue of this model, galaxies observed in near and distant regions alike have the same age on the average. The difficulties mentioned above result in additional uncertainties when testing cosmological models.

The plots in Fig. 7-2 represent the expected relation between the logarithm of the red shift and the apparent magnitude for several cosmological models [characterized by different values of the parameter $q_0 = -\ddot{R}(R \times \times H^2)^{-1}$, describing the present rate of change of the recession velocity], and the points correspond to the measured value for 18 clusters of galaxies. The validity of one of the models considered cannot be determined from this figure. Accurate observations of much fainter objects are necessary.

Counts of objects at various distances could be another observational test. If space were Euclidean and if there were no expansion, the number

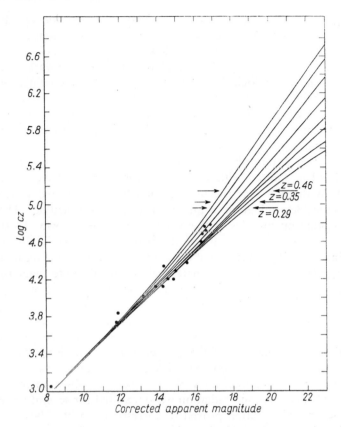

Figure 7-2. The red shift vs. the corrected apparent magnitude. The horizontal lines refer to three clusters whose magnitudes have not been determined accurately [After Sandage, *Astrophys. Journ.* **133**, 355 (1961)].

of objects seen at distances not greater than r would be proportional to r^3. However, if space is not Euclidean but has a nonvanishing curvature, the number of these objects will not be proportional to r^3 but will increase with r more or less quickly, depending on the sign of the curvature. Similarly, the expansion of the Universe will affect the dependence of this number on r. If the Universe expands, the number of distant objects in a unit volume should be greater than the number of near objects since we see near objects at a later stage, one of greater dilution. The number of objects in a unit volume will, of course, remain constant even in the event of expansion if we assume the perfect cosmological principle. Thus, counts of galaxies could be used in testing cosmological models. In this case, as before, we count objects up to a particular apparent magnitude and not up to a particular distance. Of course, here too we have all the difficulties of converting the scale of distances into the scale of apparent magnitudes, as discussed earlier. In this case as well, we are not in a position at present to determine the pertinence of any one of these models.

We shall not here present a complete survey of the various possible ways of testing cosmological models. Instead, we have confined ourselves merely to stating that in each case it is necessary to reach out to objects which are very distant and, hence, very difficult to observe.

Greater hope, as far as the choice of cosmological model is concerned, might be held out by the discovery of quasars, or in general QSO's, if these are indeed distant objects as indicated by their values of z according to Hubble's law. Objects with a red shift value of $z \approx 3$ have already been observed. With each year the number of QSO's discovered increases. In this case, too, determination of the distances entails difficulties. The values of the absolute magnitudes of these objects must be known. To this end, it is necessary to collect a wealth of observational material, and to measure the luminosities of a large number of QSO's so that statistical methods can be applied in order to evaluate their mean absolute magnitude and to detect any possible relation between the luminosities and other observable characteristics of these objects.

The discovery of blackbody background radiation discovered in the radio range a few years ago may prove to be an unexpected source of information about the past of the Universe. It was noticed that at centimetre wavelengths radio telescopes pick up radiation whose intensity exceeds the sum total of intensities of radio sources observed in the given direction. This background radiation was measured for several wavelengths and its spectral distribution proved to correspond to blackbody radiation [i.e. is described by Planck's formula; Cf. Eq. (3-93)] at a temperature of about $3°K$; it arrives isotropically from all directions and does not vary with time.

A possible interpretation of this phenomenon is to assume that the background radiation constitutes the remnants of previous stages in the evolution of the Universe. In an expanding Universe, the density of both matter and radiation (assuming the principle of conservation of mass and energy) decreases with time; however, the spectral distribution of the radiation remains a Planck distribution if it were so at any instant in the evolution, whereas all the frequencies are diminished owing to the red shift, and the maximum of the distribution moves towards the long wavelengths, which corresponds to a decrease in the temperature of the radiation. If we now go back into the past we can arrive at a state when the density and temperature of the matter were high enough for strong interaction to occur between matter and radiation. A Planck spectral distribution was established under these conditions of thermodynamic equilibrium. In still earlier phases, at a temperature of $10^{10} °K$ and somewhat higher, it was impossible for compound atomic nuclei to exist and we then had a gas of elementary particles. (We cannot say anything about earlier stages since we know too little about the behaviour of matter under such conditions.) In later periods, under particular thermal conditions, the simplest atomic nuclei of deuteron could be formed by a neutron being bound to a proton, and subsequently nuclei of tritium and helium could come into being. With a further expansion at a temperature of about 10^4 °K (plasma recombination temperature) the coupling was broken between the matter and the radiation filling the Universe, but in spite of this, its spectral distribution remained a Planck distribution, whereas the temperature decreased down to the value we now observe.

Thus observations of the background radiation of the Universe provide strong support for the evolutionary cosmological hypotheses which assume expansion of the Universe from a state in which it constituted a dense, hot, radiation-pervaded fireball of elementary particles.

Subject Index

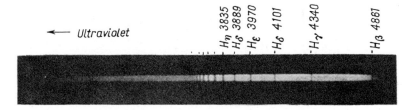

Plate 1. The spectrum of the star π_1 Cygni. A continuous and a line spectrum can be seen [Lick Observatory].

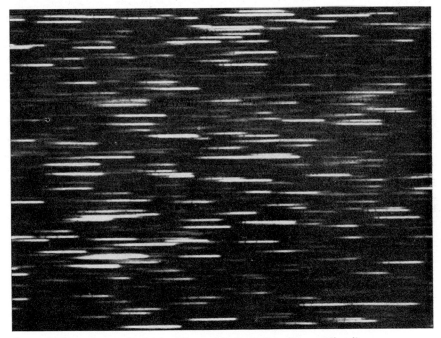

Plate 2. Stellar spectra obtained with an objective prism [From Miczaika and Sinton, *Tools of the Astronomer*, Harvard University Press, Cambridge, Mass., 1961; reprinted by permission of Harvard University Press].

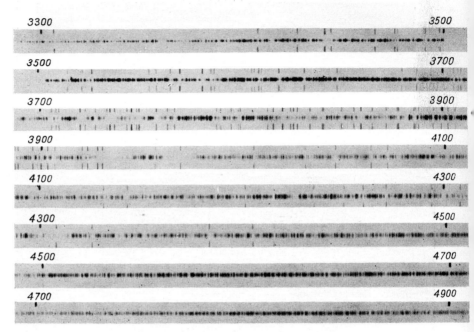

Plate 3. Spectrum of α Bootis and comparison spectra [From Miczaika and Sinton, *Tools of the Astronomer*, Harvard University Press, Cambridge, Mass., 1961; reprinted by permission of Harvard University Press].

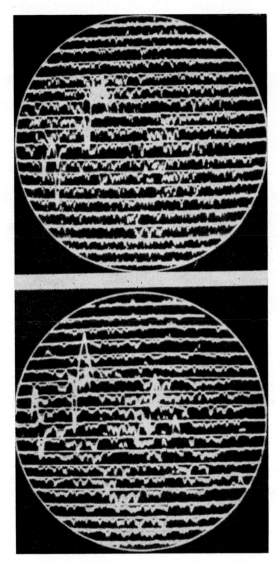

Plate 4. Solar magnetograms [Mount Wilson and Palomar Observatories].

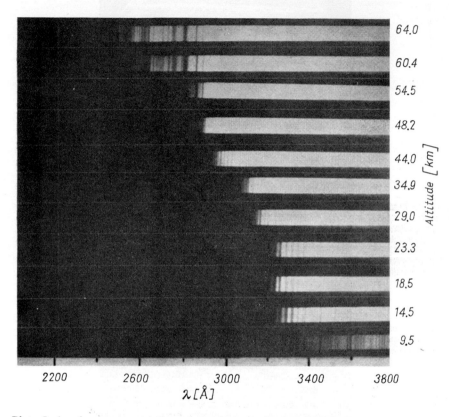

Plate 5. A solar spectrum (ultraviolet region) obtained during the flight
of a rocket to various altitudes above the Earth [Naval Research La-
boratory].

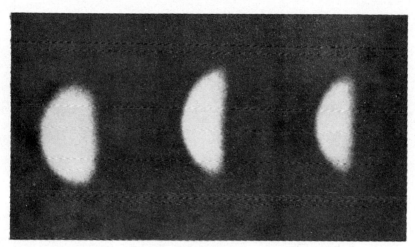

June 7, 1934   *June 11, 1934*   *June 12, 1934*

Plate 6. Mercury.

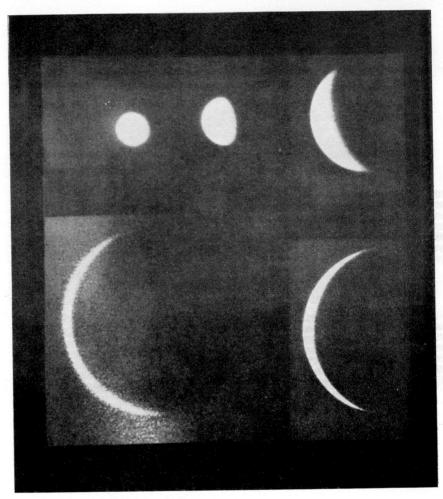

Plate 7. Venus in five different phases.

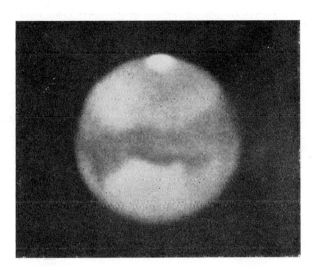

Plate 8. Mars.

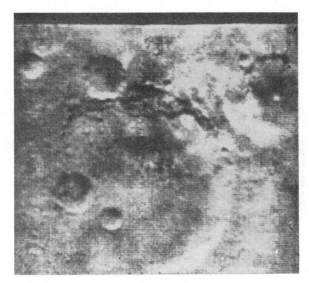

Plate 9. Part of the surface of Mars. A photograph taken by Mariner 4.

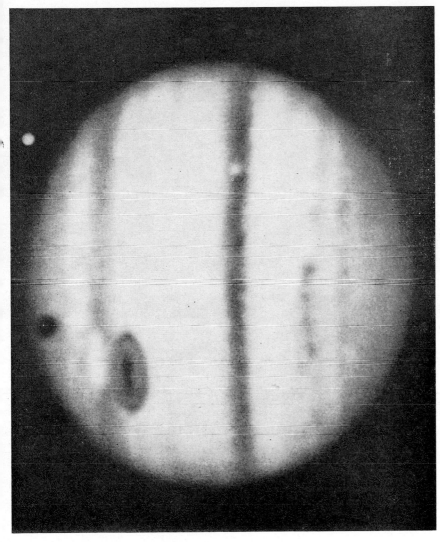

Plate 10. Jupiter [Mount Wilson and Palomar Observatories].

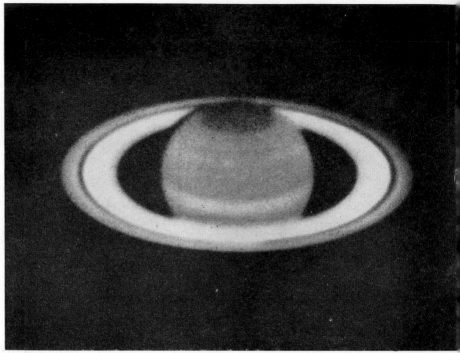

Plate 11. Saturn [Mount Wilson and Palomar Observatories].

Plate 12. The solar spectrum (green region); Fraunhöfer absorption lines against the background of the continuous spectrum [From Kiepenheuer, *The Sun*, The University of Michigan Press, Ann Arbor, Mich., 1959].

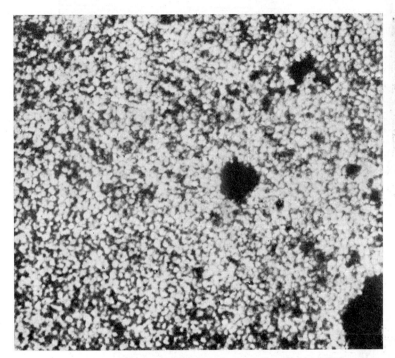

Plate 13. Photospheric granulation [Photographed by Janssen in 1885].

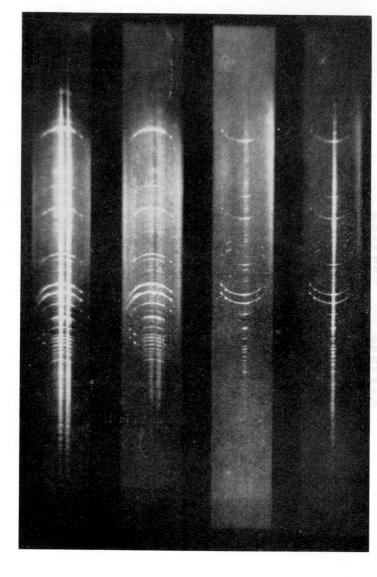

Plate 14. The chromospheric radiation spectrum during the eclipse of Aug. 31, 1932 [After Abetti].

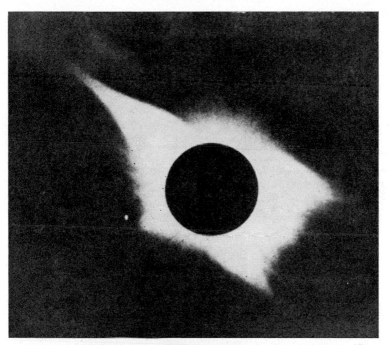

Plate 15. The solar corona on February 15, 1952 [Photographed by Bies-broeck].

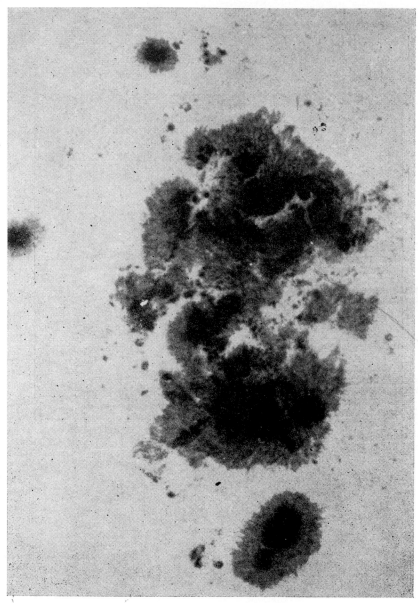

Plate 16. A group of sunspots [Mount Wilson and Palomar Observatories].

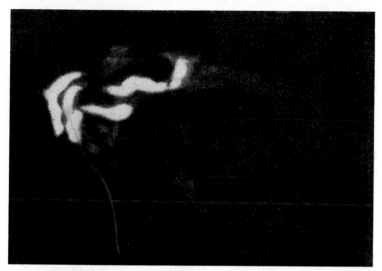

Plate 17. A spectroheliogram of a segment of the solar disk on May 10, 1949 [After Dodson].

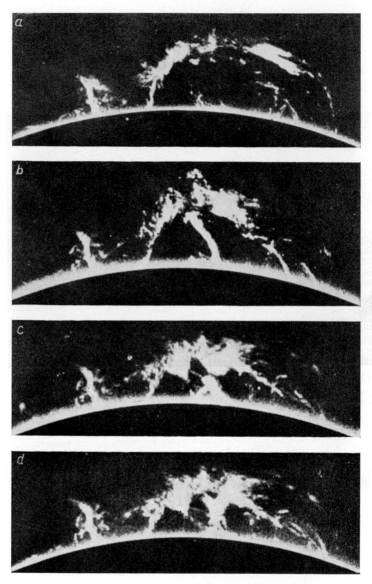

Plate 18. The development of a prominence. The time elapsed between
(a) and (d) was 40 minutes [Pic du Midi Observatory].

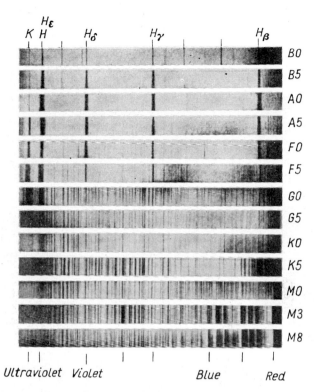

Plate 19. The spectra of stars of consecutive spectral types [From University of Michigan Observatory photographs].

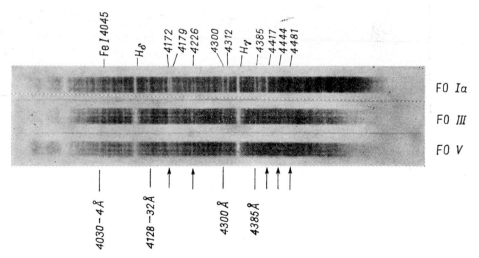

Plate 20. The spectra of type-F0 stars of consecutive classes of brightness [Yerkes Observatory].

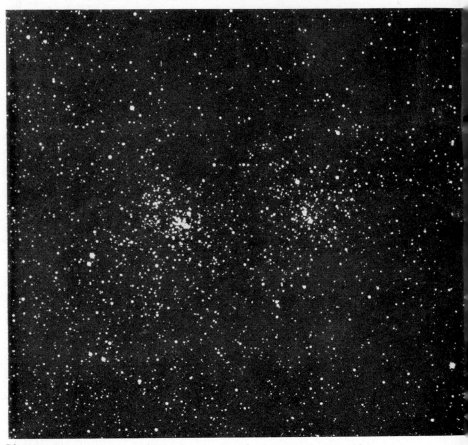

Plate 21. The double open cluster h and χ Persei [Harvard photograph].

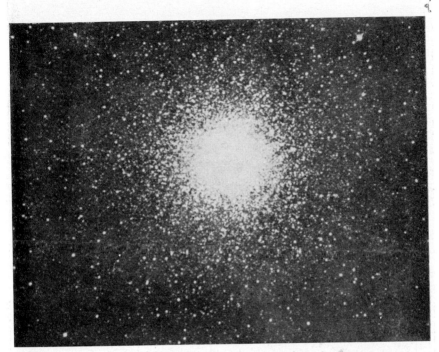

Plate 22. A globular cluster (M 3) [Mount Wilson and Palomar Observatories].

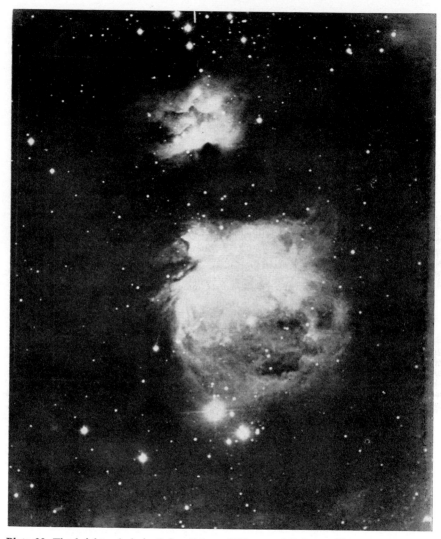

Plate 23. The bright nebula in Orion [Mount Wilson and Palomar Observatories].

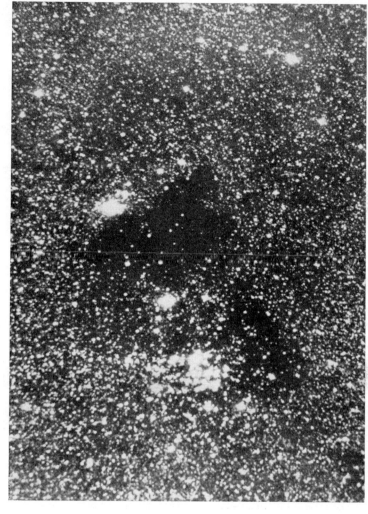

Plate 24. The dark nebula in Sagittarius [Mount Wilson and Palomar Observatories].

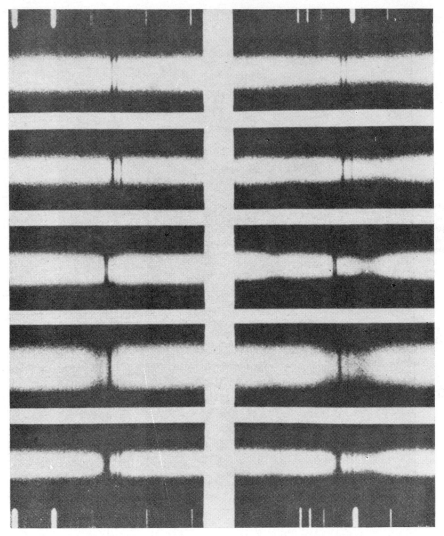

Plate 25. Interstellar lines in stellar spectra [Mount Wilson and Palomar Observatories].

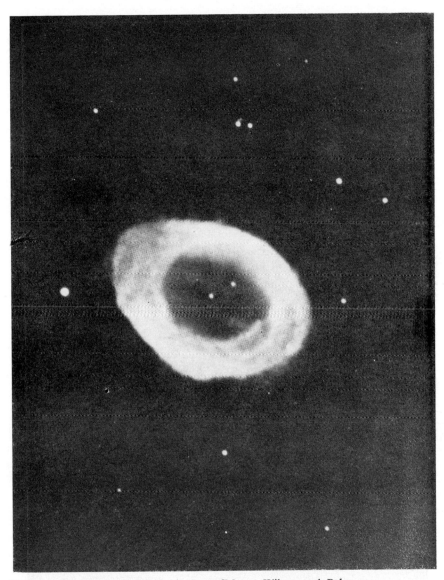

Plate 26. The planetary nebula in Lyra [Mount Wilson and Palomar Observatories].

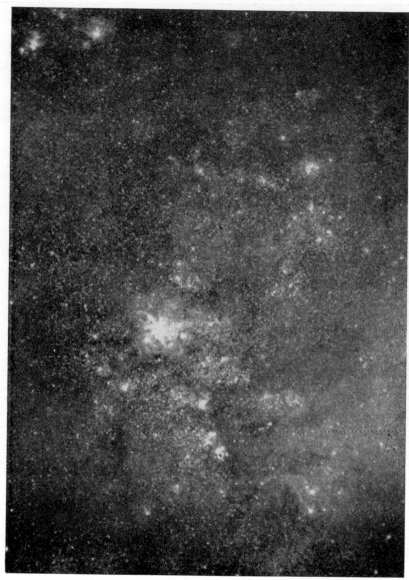

Plate 27. The Large Magellanic Cloud [Harvard photograph].

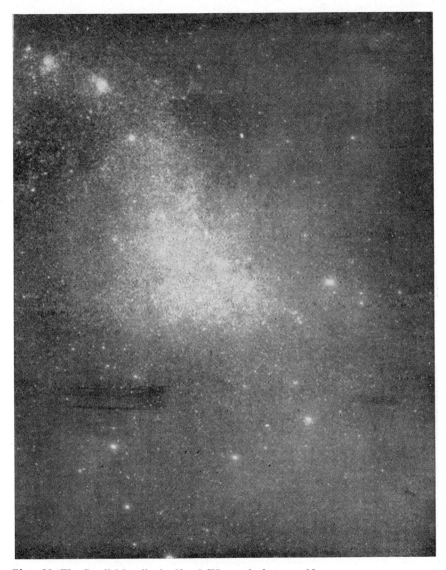

Plate 28. The Small Magellanic Cloud [Harvard photograph].

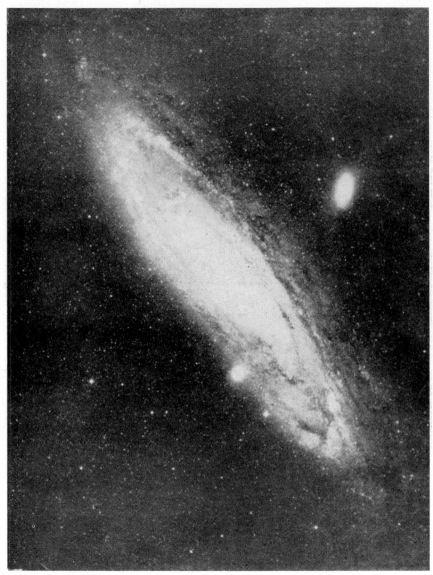

Plate 29. The Andromeda galaxy [Mount Wilson and Palomar Observatories].

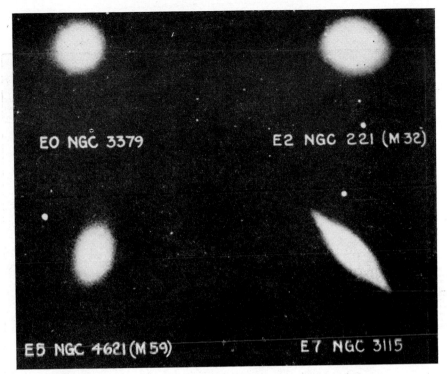

Plate 30. Elliptical galaxies [Mount Wilson and Palomar Observatories].

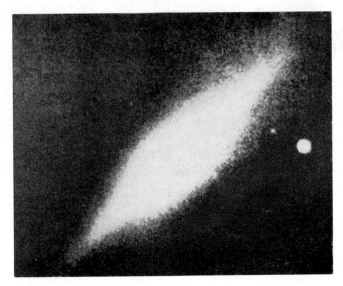

Plate 31. An *S*0 galaxy.

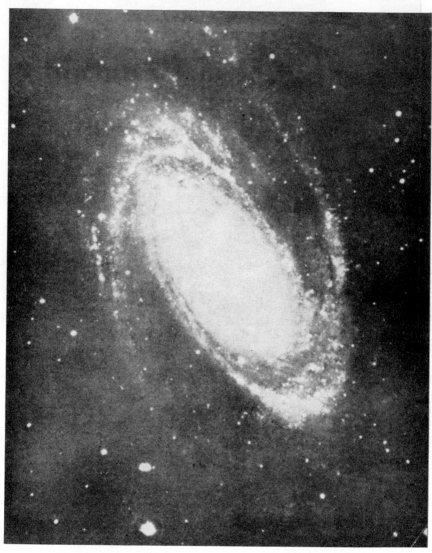

Plate 32. A spiral galaxy [Mount Wilson and Palomar Observatories].

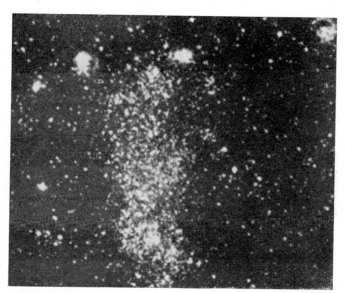

Plate 33. An irregular galaxy.

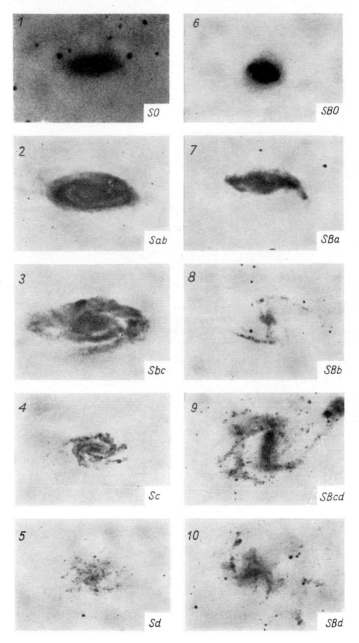

Plate 34. *S*0 and *S* galaxies according to Hubble's classification.